AGING WITH AGILITY

AGING
WITH
AGILITY

HOW ELITE ATHLETES AND
ORDINARY FOLKS EMBRACE
EXERCISE WITH AGE

MICHELLE PANNOR
SILVER

Columbia University Press   *New York*

Columbia University Press
Publishers Since 1893
New York   Chichester, West Sussex

Library of Congress Cataloging-in-Publication Data
Names: Silver, Michelle Pannor, author.
Title: Aging with agility : how elite athletes and ordinary folks
embrace exercise with age / Michelle Pannor Silver.
Other titles: How elite athletes and ordinary folks
embrace exercise with age
Description: First edition. | New York : Columbia University Press,
[2025] | Includes index.
Identifiers: LCCN 2025008347 | ISBN 9780231219730 (hardback) |
ISBN 9780231219747 (trade paperback) |
ISBN 9780231562874 (ebook)
Subjects: LCSH: Physical fitness for older people. |
Aging. | Health. | Quality of life.
Classification: LCC GV482.6 .S53 2025 |
DDC 613.7/0446—dc23/eng/20250417

Cover design: Milenda Nan Ok Lee
Cover art: Michelle Pannor Silver

GPSR Authorized Representative: Easy Access System Europe,
Mustamäe tee 50, 10621 Tallinn, Estonia, gpsr.requests@easproject.com

CONTENTS

1 On Your Mark   1

2 Focus   33

3 Confidence   57

4 Motivation   85

5 Resilience   110

6 Optimism   133

7 Commitment   156

8 Rules for the Endgame   180

Methodological Appendix   201

Notes   213

Index   229

CONTENTS

AGING WITH AGILITY

1

ON YOUR MARK

Be yourself; everyone else is already taken.
—Oscar Wilde

For most of human history, life expectancy has been around thirty-five years. Now, global life expectancy is over seventy years. Yes, there have always been people who have lived well beyond seventy years; however, there has never been this many people living this long. In less than two hundred years, we have more than doubled our life expectancy—this is a most remarkable achievement of human civilization. However, living longer requires that we spend more time thinking about how we want to live our later years. It is the rare person who lives more than three or four decades without allocating time to the physical maintenance of their own body, financial planning, and thinking about how to avoid pain and suffering. While there have always been people who lived to the century mark, striking differences are emerging as more of us live nearer that milestone. Some of us have aged beyond our chronological years, while others are in the best shapes of their lives. Some of us are in pursuit of growing older without showing any of the signs of aging.

The number of master athletes, those athletes who have highly specific knowledge about their sport and participate at an age that is above what is considered the typical age of peak performance, has grown exponentially. There are more master athletes competing today than the total number of master athletes who have lived and died before. As international sports competition times and ages have increased, so have the number and cost of health-care treatments that can help us live longer lives. Some of us inhabit bodies that demonstrate the limits of human physical capabilities; others are living longer lives with multiple chronic conditions and other traits that in previous times would have prevented longevity.

For many of us, our last few years are or will be very different from what our parents and grandparents experienced. Some of us have had the opportunity to watch our parents react to the ways their parents aged. This influences our own ideas about whether we want to be providers of care for our parents or ensure there is an assisted-living facility in mind and an elder-care plan in place. Others come from families where members died younger, so our images of the later stages of life are less clear or based on movies, books, and other influences. This book asks you to think about how you imagine spending the last few chapters of your life. It is an exploration of a range of perspectives and ways of thinking about exercise, aging, movement, and functional abilities over time.

The heart of this book is a series of chapters that feature the stories of people whose life experiences embody the notion of aging with agility. They have different orientations toward exercise, but there is much to be learned from listening to their lived experiences. As their stories illustrate, aging is no simple endeavor. It is my hope that attending to how others think about aging and exercise, over time and from a range of different orientations, will evoke an interest that helps you formulate your own relationship to movement and ultimately your own rules for the endgame.

I embarked on this book with the hypothesis that athletes and people in the world of sports would have unique insights regarding exercising with age. I found this to be true, but not always in ways that I had predicted. Among the people featured within these chapters are those who represented their country at an Olympic Games, some of whom became professional coaches. Others never participated in sport. Some live with chronic pain or chronic disease. One had polio as a child and has successfully thrived through decades of mobility challenges. One lives a very sedentary life and has severe mobility issues. Still, within this group are people who came to be in the best shape of their lives in their seventies and eighties. I interviewed each person over the course of approximately a decade to learn their stories in relation to their perceptions about aging and exercise over the years. Each reflected on the time they have lived, how their bodies have served them, and how they have taken care of their bodies.[1]

This book gives embodiment (the realization of how interactions with social and physical environments influence our physical and emotional well-being) an important place in understanding what it is like to transition into mature adulthood. It takes a phenomenological approach to thinking about senescence, or the process of growing old. Corporeality, or the fact of existing as a physical body, can be understood in the context of aging and embodiment as reflecting the social context and cultural beliefs about aging that we hear, learn, and incorporate. Epigenetics is the influence of one's environment on gene expression, and embodied aging can be understood as the ways that our environments shape our perceptions about aging—and in turn how we age.[2]

My goal in interviewing each of the people in this book was to learn about their perspectives on and experiences with aging and exercise. Over the course of speaking with each person for approximately a decade, I learned there are many ways our perceptions about aging influence how we take care of our bodies. Some searched for the fountain of youth through cosmetic surgery, creams, injections, and hair dye; others pursued drugs and medications to ameliorate their aliments. A few avoided exercise entirely, and others found that exercise enhanced their transition to later life stages. Each presented different ways of thinking about mobility, functionality, and physical limitations.

It would be great to have an oracle to advise us on our optimal path, particularly during uncertain times. Alas, this book does not hold any special powers to predict anyone's future and makes no claims about the optimal body type or ideal exercise routine for your body. Instead, it is about perceptions about aging and exercise. By presenting in-depth examples, this book simply asks you to consider whether and how you might age with agility.

AGING WITH AGILITY

Agility is the ability to move quickly and easily. Aging is the accumulation of diverse changes that take place in the cells and tissues over time, all of which increase the risk of disease and death. If being mobile and independent for as long as possible is a goal of aging, being agile is the prized goal of aging. We begin aging from the moment we are born. Much of aging is involuntary and out of our control. Some of our cells age faster than others; some of us age faster than others. Yet as simple as it is to define and experience aging, it remains a complex process. A great many things can be done to ameliorate or alter the aging process, yet none is more likely to enhance your health than exercise.

The question of whether exercise equates to health is contentious. Exercise and health are what economists might describe as endogenous because each concept is a predictor of each outcome. In other words, are we healthy because we exercise? Or are we able to exercise because we are healthy? Both are true. It important to acknowledge up-front that some people live in chronic pain, with chronic seizures, or with chronic disabilities, to name a few examples. And this means that exercise and aging are significantly more complex. It also means that we should consider how best to support complex bodies when creating efforts to embrace aging with agility.

What it means to be healthy seems to be becoming an ever-tougher question. The World Health Organization (WHO) defines health as a state of complete physical, mental, and social well-being.[3] The WHO challenges biomedical models of disease, which suggest that disease, disability, or illness render a person less healthy. While the main aim of the biomedical model of disease is to understand the mechanisms causing disease and thus diagnose and treat it, mixed outcomes have arisen from this method of portraying and studying health. A strict biomedical model of health not only fails to account for lived experiences, particularly those that include experiences of disability, chronic disease, chronic pain, and multiple morbidities, it also overlooks the ways that economic, political, social, environmental, and psychological context affect health. More holistic and thorough understandings of health consider physical or mental health, as well as occupational, intellectual, spiritual, social, and emotional health.[4]

There are many ways to refer to people at different stages in the aging process. "Toddlers," "youth," "teenagers," and "young adults" are a few terms used to refer to those in the early stages of life. In the later stages, the terms we use are somewhat contentious. At many points in history, the words to describe later life have evoked negative associations, including physical decline and economic hardship. Mature bodies are unfortunately often depicted in ways that aim to shock and attract revulsion. Some aspects of getting old tend to be depicted with a focus on the negative and disgusting, which in turn are held up as justification for trepidation. The commode in the bedroom must be regularly emptied and cleaned. The skin folds around the bottom require assistance to be cleaned properly. Toes cannot be reached and thus they require assistance, even if they smell bad because urine sometimes makes its way down the leg on the way back to bed. Hair that cannot be brushed becomes matted, and this is to say nothing of eyebrows that once were tweezed regularly or nails that once were painted.[5]

Before the turn of the last century, mature characters tended to be vilified when they were included in literature and film. Think of Scrooge or the "wicked old witch" or any character depicting a person in later stages of life in horror films. There are reasons to be cautious in labeling someone based on their chronological age. Although it is not specific, the term "mature adult" can be helpful for distinguishing the decades of life that occur as we approach one hundred. I use it throughout this book because of its lack of specificity and because we associate maturity with life experience.[6]

Health and aging are inextricably linked. Most people advance in years by virtue of having good health. Aging is the passing of time, the accumulation of experiences, and the experience of acquiring wear and tear on the body. Gerontology is the study of aging, and it draws from many fields, including biology, psychology, sociology, health policy, history, economics, and others. Advanced age is the number-one risk factor for most chronic disease, particularly when combined with sedentary behavior. Aging is associated with decline in the functioning of many of our senses, including sight and hearing. For some people, it is also associated with declines in activities of daily life, frailty, and disability. For others, it is associated with an increased interest in taking good care of the body and engaging in activities to promote health.

The term "senescence" refers to the process of deteriorating with age. Both aging and senescence occur throughout the life course. One way to think about distinguishing the two is to consider that the number of senescent cells in our bodies increase with age. Because our cells are the most basic units of life, responsible for all of life's processes, this fact implies that we deteriorate with age. For all the ways our cells and organs decline with age, the aged body is the precursor to death—we may resist this reality by trying to make sense of, ameliorate, or ignore the changes that take place in our maturing bodies.

In gerontology, time is important. Time marks the progress of existence. We measure our progress with the passing of time, and our measures of time hold us accountable. The ways our bodies develop and are shaped or become out of shape are influenced by the passage of time and the way we manage our time. In addition to being both a noun and a verb, time is also an excuse. The main reason people give for not exercising is that they don't have enough time. Another is that they cannot afford to exercise. Societies around the world must note these challenges with finding ways to support people so that they can make time to stretch intentionally or move in the way their unique bodies allow.

AGELESS AGING

We are constrained by time from the moment we are conceived. From the age categories that limit our participation in a given sport to the age-related changes that slow us down to the stopwatch that brutally imposes winners and losers, timing is everything. We win, we lose, we live, and we die in ways that are marked by time. Our perceptions of time and what we each think it means to be a certain age influence the stories our bodies tell about how we have passed our days. This is because our perceptions about aging can determine how we care for our bodies and minds and because our understandings of time influence how we use our time.

Understandings of youthful beauty suggest that gray hair, wrinkles, and receding hairlines are our enemies. There are a great many pressures in society to figure out how to age by not becoming or not appearing old. The mature body can be viewed as a distinct biological entity, associated with remorse for what it once was. For those hoping to die before they grow old, there are reasons to try to slow down senescence. Arguably the most popularized depiction of the aged body is the medicalized body. In the medicalized body, anything that does not function optimally is diagnosed as subpar, something to be remedied. It is therefore scrutinized for signs of decline and malfunction. This scrutiny can be overwhelming for many of us who live in bodies that no longer function the way they used to. There are also many of us who live in bodies that never functioned the way the medical gaze and much of society assumes they should.[7]

Society's obsession with looking youthful is not new. Ponce de León is credited with seeking out the fountain of youth in the early 1500s. Recent decades have witnessed a proliferation in medical interventions, cosmetic surgeries, and pharmaceuticals for weight loss that make it possible for us to feel younger—and in some cases to live longer. Current trends among mature adults feature body work practices that aim to craft faces and bodies that mimic those of people in very early adulthood. It is no secret that skin care products generate billions annually in commercial markets around the world. The number of antiaging surgical procedures has skyrocketed dramatically since the baby boomers entered the stages of mature adulthood. Injections and procedures that aim to promote youthful aging are on the rise.[8]

The pursuit of a long life has taken on new forms as more of us are living longer. One way out of old age is to manage, control, or hide visible signs and signals of agedness. Pharmaceutical drugs that help regulate our bodily processes make it possible to avoid the consequences of cardiovascular disease that killed off earlier generations. In particular, statin drugs that lower levels of cholesterol and triglycerides in the blood have reduced mortality rates dramatically. And what could be better than simply taking a pill and living longer? However, if the goal is no longer simply to live longer but to live longer healthier, then we must keep moving our bodies in whatever manner they can move.[9]

The notion of subjective aging means taking time into your own hands, living according to how you feel, and making your own interpretations of what it means to move and function in meaningful ways. This book is largely about people who have focused on feeling good as opposed to feeling a certain age. Our ability to understand how our bodies change with age, how we are motivated to change or maintain our habits, and how we analyze and learn from our losses and life transitions is one of the many unique traits that distinguish us from other living beings. We humans have the ability to make conscious decisions to change our patterns of behavior if or when our habits lead us down suboptimal paths.

Remember, how we age depends on a host of factors. One important way of explaining differences in our health by age is by considering social determinants of health, such as the environments in which we live and how these affect our physical functioning, well-being, risks, and health outcomes. Our bodies function differently at birth, for instance, and our aging is shaped by the circumstances we grow up in and the context in which we live our lives. For example, economic status and social class shape the opportunities we have to play sports, which sports we play, and whether we exercise at all. The places we are born and where we live determine whether we have access to essential resources like health care and emotional support. Our physical environment, including access to clean air, clean water, and safe spaces to exercise also influences how we age.[10]

Economic analyses underscore the benefit of exercise to society in numeric terms: more people engaging in more exercise reduces expenses associated with chronic disease treatment. Exercise is good for society, and it's good for *you*, too. Among other things, regular exercise strengths muscles and bones, enhances circulation, improves mood, promotes better sleep, aids with maintaining weight, and can be a way to connect socially.[11]

"Physical activity" is an umbrella term that includes any body movement that requires energy expenditure and is produced by the engagement of skeletal muscles. Exercise, on the other hand, is a type of physical activity done to maintain or improve fitness that involves intentional and repetitive body movement. Exercise is a means to becoming physically fit—a controversial term because determining what constitutes a fit person is subjective and differs over time, region, and culture. Generally speaking, however, "fitness" can be defined as a set of attributes that people acquire and that relates to their ability to engage in physical activity. Fitness encompasses components that are health related, skill related, and physiological. Another term to keep in mind is "body work," which describes the regular upkeep and maintenance we do for our bodies—everything from brushing our teeth to washing and moving our bodies. It is hard to understate the importance of exercise as body work.

Body work, exercise, and fitness are not without controversy. Exercise is associated with the promotion of thin and youthful appearances in ways that body-shame and fail to accept a range of body types and lifestyles. Its promotion has been criticized as an elitist and ableist mechanism for enhancing health among the wealthy. Further complicating the concept of exercise is the fact that most health-care professionals receive little to no training about exercise.[12]

Some bodies can't expend energy in ways that other bodies can. We are each born with different types of bodies and varying degrees of physical ability. The extent to which our bodies can be perceived as medicalized versus malleable determines the extent to which we, as individuals and as a society, shift toward becoming agents who embrace aging with agility. Certain congenital conditions prohibit forms of movement that many of us take for granted. Illness, accidents, congenital conditions, and conditions that develop along the life course can limit the control we have over our bodily movements. Our bodies differ, and our physical abilities change with age. Thus, when the terms "agility," "movement," "exercise," and "fitness" are used here, it is with the understanding that we cannot and will not all move in the same ways. While it is important to note that, every year, over 5 million premature deaths are directly linked with sedentary behaviors, it is equally important to avoid narratives that blame rather than encourage people to move in the ways that they are able. "Exercise," "physical activity," and "fitness" are relatively easy to define, but it is less clear why and how some of us come to incorporate exercise in our lives, while others avoid it like the plague.

PERCEPTIONS OF TIME AND AGING

Time is both fluid and fixed. Sometimes we feel like we have all the time in the world. Sometimes time really doesn't matter— like when you are falling in love or doing something you consider to be most important in the world. Because our world is largely governed by rules around time, however, time is crucial in many aspects of our lives.

The concept of standard time emerged in the United States in 1883. It was needed to create common schedules for railroads. Until then, cities had kept their own local time, which was often determined by the sun or moon and differed from place to place. In Britain, too, prior to railway impositions, town and church clocks set the standard and citizens simply set their own pocket timepieces according to the chimes. Soon, technology allowed for synchronization around the world and beyond. One hundred years ago, it would have been inconceivable to be able to measure time at the precise level we are able today. Because of smartphones and wearable devices, time is never far from our minds.

Timing became important to sport, especially in Olympic competition, starting in the late eighteenth century. It was necessary to measure precisely how much faster one athlete was relative to another. Even so, stopwatches, or timing devices that could measure units of time less than one second, were not developed until the early nineteenth century. And the operation of stopwatches by official timekeepers was subject to human error until the Olympics went electronic in 1964 at the Tokyo Summer Games. Four years later, in Mexico City, pressure-sensitive touch pads were introduced in swimming events, and false-start detectors came into use in track and field at the 1984 Olympic Games in Los Angeles. The 1996 Olympic Games in Atlanta, Georgia, brought GPS and radio transponders to cycling events.

Now, about thirty years later, a single pixel's distance between two competitors can distinguish a medal ranking.

Aging moves by a different, more individual clock. Our chronological age often tells us little beyond when our next birthday will be. Some people consider fifty a milestone birthday that marks a new stage of life—that as an "older adult"— while others consider fifty just the start of adulthood. Others cringe at the very idea of aging and will barely utter the dreaded words "old" and "older." Reviews of the literature indicate that older people feel younger than they actually are and that positive expressions of aging correspond with better health outcomes. Cultural stereotypes about the negative aspects of our own aging are associated with worse health outcomes later in life. At all ages, those who believe that we become less attractive, more depressed, angry, or upset with age are less likely to live longer. Researchers and policymakers around the world are shifting away from framing aging as a time of decline and toward thinking about aging as a time to prioritize quality of life.[13]

From our earliest civilizations, we have been on a quest to learn how to live a long and healthy life. Human survival has always depended on figuring out what foods to avoid, how best to avoid injury or death, and what sorts of shelter would provide the best protection. Many of us today eagerly seek information on what exercises maximize muscle and bone development, what sorts of homes are the most conducive to growing old. The United Nations (UN) has created the Active Ageing Index (AAI) as a way of measuring and comparing the engagement of mature adults. The AAI measures mature adults' potential for healthy and active living through a composite of indicators, including participation in paid employment, physical exercise, caregiving, engagement in social and learning activities, and other factors that influence independence across different countries. These measures attest to the value of keeping active in our later years. They also help us question what it means to have an actively engaged mature population. Although the quest to learn how we can avoid or embrace aging is not novel, the need to address the challenges that arise with a growing population of mature adults has never been more essential to our survival.[14]

ALL'S FAIR IN LOVE, WAR, AND SPORTS

Elite athletes illustrate the limits of what we are physically capable of as humans. The way we focus our attention and resources on them while they are in their prime and then discard them once they step down from the podium, however, exemplifies some of issues that we ought to confront as we try to live long healthy lives. Following athletes through their athletic retirement transitions, listening to them when they are no longer in their prime, is valuable. Their experiences can teach us many things, like the fact that none of us know what sorts of injuries or defeat lurk around the corner and that with time we can learn to recalibrate our sense of self in ways that are sustainable. Three of the people who shared their stories for this book were elite athletes approximately four decades prior to our interviews; two became athletic coaches, one became a master athlete, and each had unique struggles with exercise. Their perceptions about aging and exercise differed, but they shared common understandings about the level of commitment required to be an elite athlete and unique perspectives on how to care for an aging body.

Our collective fascination remains strong when it comes to the elite athletes who illustrate the limits of our physical potential as humans—look no further than the multibillion-dollar world of sports. Attention and resources are focused on athletes while they are in their prime, with intense scrutiny on speed, strength, and agility. Once our favored athletes reach the peak of their careers and step down from the podium, we abandon and discard them as we often move on to more youthful hopefuls.

Unlike love and war, sports have rules and the expectation of fairness. Winners are typically determined by speed, jumping or throwing the farthest, or making the most goals. In every sport, there are elements that are not just based on luck but are simply unfair. Some athletes receive better coaching. Some have better facilities, safer equipment, trusted coaches, and greater resources to support their training; some even have access to performance-enhancing drugs. Victory is often associated with youth, speed, and dominance, all of which can stem from vast inequalities throughout an athlete's life.

Whether you live in a favela or the most affluent neighborhood around, you understand speed: speed knows no boundaries. Speed creates heroes. In our excitement to celebrate winning in sports, we push athletes to be faster, more flexible, and stronger at all costs. We often fail, however, to question our obsession with speed to the detriment of individual athletes. Our obsession with speed is also counter to our collective social interest in aging sustainably.

Elite athletes are recognized for achieving seemingly impossible physical standards, but sports are a business. When athletes are no longer in their prime, when an athlete slows down because of injury, decline, or aging, they are often cast aside for newer, younger, and stronger replacements. The ageism they experience is striking because it frequently occurs at such a young age.

Ageism, or discrimination based on age, is all around us. Judgments that aging is bad are reflected in the abundance of antiaging, reverse aging, and aging defying products. Many of us are desperate to hide the signs of our own aging because we have come to see time as the enemy. There is perhaps no group of people more likely to see time as the enemy than elite athletes. In sports, timing is nearly everything. Olympic sports that used to measure to the tenth of a minute now measure to the tenth of a second. One of Michael Phelps's gold medals was won by one hundredth of a second—literally less than the blink of an eye.

Elite sports require a set of traits and skills that must be identified and developed early. Sports favor able-bodied, committed, and coordinated youth. To be an elite athlete, training generally begins within the first decade of life and involves an intense level of commitment maintained over years. Most elite athletes clock well over the ten thousand hours of practice said to create mastery. Sport specialization, or intense year-round training in a single sport, has been promoted as necessary to achieve elite levels and is generally initiated in early childhood with the support of parents and diligent training from coaches.[15]

There are numerous benefits to early and intense sports participation. Early athletic development helps kids develop balance and coordination. Sports can be social and promote an active lifestyle. Sports teach kids to focus and develop accountability to their teammates. The many favorable traits associated with sports and athleticism include those that are included in the chapter titles of this book: focus, confidence, motivation, resilience, optimism, and commitment.

On the other hand, early and intense sports participation can cause anxiety; expose kids to bullying from fellow players and coaches; and lead to high rates of injury, pressure, burnout, and even a desire *not* to play as the athlete ages. In the United States, most kids quit sports by age thirteen, and only slightly over 20 percent of men and just under 20 percent of women play any sport as adults. Nearly everyone who has played a sport has experienced some form of minor injury. However, for elite athletes, particularly those in hockey, football, basketball, and soccer, injuries can be debilitating, life threatening, and lifelong. They can become chronic conditions, and they can contribute to physical limitations with age.

Another concern with organized sports is that, while it keeps players physically active, it is otherwise a generally sedentary experience for nearly everyone else. Most sports fans sit while they watch the game. It has been suggested that events like the Olympics inspire people to take up sports, but the evidence suggests that watching sports, on TV or live at a venue, has no significant impact on the promotion of physical activity and is linked to significantly higher incidence of sedentary behavior.[16]

Another problem is that we invest billions of public dollars in state-of-the-art athletic facilities, yet these facilities are regularly abandoned in the wake of international sports events. Investment in infrastructure that would support those among us with the physical limitations that can be associated with aging or possessing a body that functions differently tend to be low and unusual. Many major cities have expensive outdoor gyms in parks and along walking paths that are almost never used. Most of our cities lack basic necessities in dense areas, like wheelchair ramps, accessible public washrooms, clear pathways, and elevators, that are essential to movement in daily life for many people. Nonurban regions tend to fare even worse when it comes to accessible public space.

The body keeps track of lack of care in ways that have a plethora of implications for the individual, for families, and for the public systems responsible for providing care. As more of us live longer, more of us are living longer with multiple chronic conditions and with significant physical mobility limitations, but there is also a subset of elite athletes breaking world records in every age group. Master athletes start at thirty-five years old (the same age that cardiovascular issues tend to become a significant cause of morbidity) to compete in five-year age brackets past one hundred years, so that the youngest competitors are between 35 and 39 and the oldest grouping is 105 to 109 years old.

The last several decades have seen a continual increase in the number of these master athletes. The first U.S. National Senior Games in 1987 had 2,500 participants; in 2022, there were more than 12,000 participants. The New York City Marathon has seen the number of athletes over the age of 50 increase by well over 100 percent. Many master athletes are experienced competitors who participate because they are eager to continue in their sport once they have aged out of more youthful competitions. Others return after extended periods of inactivity. Still others find their way later in life, like Olga Kotelko, a remarkable master athlete who started in sports at seventy years old.[17]

With higher participation rates, we have observed better performance and greater records set by people in older age groups. New training methods, master athlete coaching, nutritional strategies, and generally enhanced overall physical conditions among mature adults are also factors that contribute to impressive records emerging among master athletes. Because maximal oxygen consumption, or the maximum rate of oxygen consumption attainable during physical exertion, tends to decrease around age thirty-five, master athletes hold key insights for our ability to maintain physical performance with age.[18]

A BRIEF HISTORY OF EXERCISE

For much of human history, fitness has been linked to health and survival. In addition to work, social, religious, and cultural activities, exercise has generally been recognized as key to a good, long life. For the first humans, strength and mobility were developed through necessity-driven daily practices required to secure food and safe shelter. Across Africa, for instance, physical activity has been a consistent and critical feature of daily life from the earliest records of human history; ancient Egyptians, for example, placed great value on spine flexibility. Chinese descriptions from as early as 3,000 BCE portray physical activity as essential to the principle of human harmony, and physical inactivity as associated with internal blockages and organ malfunction.

The Old Testament also promotes the value of fitness and its role in defense among warriors. Both Hindu and Buddhist philosophies prioritized spirituality over physical development, but body control became an important keystone in hatha yoga, and martial arts developed from basic principles linked to these early religions. Starting around 10,000 BCE, the agricultural revolution saw the transition for humans from hunter-gatherers to farmers, which meant that more people began to engage in a more limited range of repetitive movements.

During the Roman Empire, all Roman citizens between seventeen and sixty years of age were expected to keep fit enough to train and serve in the military. Aristotle suggests that the first Olympic Games, in 776 BCE, were developed to showcase the practical movements that were helpful in wars. Toward the end of the Roman Empire, military training became the predominant means of physical training. Preparing for battle helped men develop muscle. Soon athletic competitions and sports cultures developed in societies around the world.

In addition to military training and sports, the Common Era celebrated the beauty of the human body in ways that embraced physical training as part of a complete education. Being fit was a critical component of being a well-rounded and well-regarded person. In the Dark Ages, however, the body became sinful in much of the world, and the focus of training shifted to the mind. The Renaissance revived interest in the body and led to the development of physical education. Starting around 1760, with the industrial revolution, manual forms of production transitioned to machine-based industry. The workweek decreased from seventy hours in 1860 to the point now where forty hours or less is the norm for full-time work in much of the Western world. The industrial revolution changed the way people worked, moved many people away from rural areas, established urban centers, and shifted the way people moved. Factories and industrial warehouses were largely filled with people who sat for prolonged periods behind machines and moved relatively less than previous generations had.

As workdays became more sedentary, physical movement had to become more intentional. In many parts of Europe, being fit became a civic duty. First circulated in 1859, Charles Darwin's notion of the "survival of the fittest" boosted interest in physical fitness. Fitness was important in early twentieth-century Germany when Friedrich Han developed ideas about physical education that spread around much of the world. By the late 1800s, the general hygiene movement had begun in the United States with the support of physicians who were influenced by these European ideas and promoted exercise programs in the schools.

The world wars of the twentieth century also placed great importance on physical abilities and motivated people to get in shape in the name of national vigor. Men who were deemed not healthy enough could not fight for their countries, and women who were not strong enough could not keep farms and factories going on the home front. In the wake of World War II, many countries established universal health-care systems to improve general health and devoted attention to developing healthier citizens by formalizing physical education programs in schools.

In the 1960s, North America witnessed a fitness revolution. The American College of Sports Medicine (ACSM) was established, and the influential book *Aerobics* was first published. The study of physical activity, epidemiology, was established, leading to the scientific collection of evidence linking exercise and good health. This led to the development of guidelines for types and recommended amounts of physical activity. By the 1970s, the American Heart Association (AHA) had published an exercise testing and training handbook, and the ACSM had issued its guidelines for the intensity, duration, mode, and frequency of exercise needed to be physically fit. As we neared the twenty-first century, however, many of the physical education programs established after World War II were removed or limited because of budget cuts. Thus came a shift toward the privatization of fitness.[19]

Ideas about what it means to be fit and how to exercise in order to illustrate your fitness can now be found in magazines, in film, on television, and primarily on social media. Looking to the United States in particular, we can note a significant shift toward profit-driven fitness, which is illustrated through fads that demonstrate "ideal" physiques and ways to achieve them. One such fad, emblematic of the fitness revolution, featured jogging and Jazzercise. Fitness fads eventually became features of private sports training facilities and elite gyms with private trainers. The fitness movement has more recently embraced home gym equipment, modern fitness apps, and omnipresent wearable devices.[20]

Every city around the world has at least one gym or fitness studio that offers a range of ways that you can pay to exercise. There is no shortage of books or online resources to advise you about the best way to get in shape. Around the world, national guidelines tell us how often and how much exercise we should get. And yet much of the world's people do not adhere to basic physical activity guidelines. It is unlikely that any given person can simply read a guideline and feel convinced to change their behaviors. Forming healthy habits is a process.

YOU MIGHT NOT WANT TO SIT DOWN FOR THIS

You might have heard that "sitting is the new smoking," that a sedentary lifestyle is now understood as a lifestyle choice that will drastically reduce your health and potentially your life span. Little or no physical activity is, by definition, what makes people sedentary, and it is linked with chronic conditions that can make it more difficult to be physically active. The treatment of chronic conditions is expensive. Plus, being sedentary is associated with depression and lack of engagement with life.[21]

Sedentary behavior is almost nonexistent among young children; well over 90 percent of younger children in the United States are considered physically active. Yet over 25 percent of U.S. adults are not active at all, and more than 60 percent do not engage in the amount of weekly activity recommended by the Centers for Disease Control and Prevention (CDC). Women are more likely than men to be less physically active, as are mature adults relative to younger adults, less affluent people relative to those with greater wealth, people who are visible minorities relative to white people, and people with less family and social support relative to those with more. Keep in mind, however, that not all bodies respond similarly to regular physical activity. Because of genetic differences and hereditary predispositions, some people show greater improvements in fitness, for example, by developing muscle tone quicker, relative to others in the same activity program.

Whether you are sitting at a desk, behind the wheel, or in front of a screen, sitting is bad for your posture and your waistline. Sitting for long periods is associated with increased blood pressure and body fat. Large numbers of sedentary adults reaching mature adulthood poses several concerns for societies around the world. Sedentary behavior is linked with chronic conditions, such as those that last at least a year and tend to require ongoing medical attention, like heart disease and diabetes. These chronic conditions tend to limit your ability to perform the basic activities of daily living (ADLs), including the things you need to do regularly like getting dressed, bathing, cooking, getting in and out of a chair, or going to the toilet on your own.

Chronic conditions are the leading causes of death in nearly every part of the world, partly because we have shifted away, almost universally, from infectious disease as the major cause of world mortality. We are more likely to live past childhood and into late adulthood, and so we are more likely to die of chronic conditions. The demographic transition or shift caused by reductions in childhood mortality from infectious disease has led to reductions in fertility rates. As more children survive childhood, women give birth to fewer children on average, and a higher percentage of the population reaches adulthood. Globalization and urbanization have led to an epidemiological transition whereby health-care needs have shifted from infectious diseases to chronic or degenerative diseases.[22]

As more people live longer, the number of people living with *multiple* chronic conditions has skyrocketed. A relevant concern here is higher health-care costs. The CDC estimates that chronic conditions account for 90 percent of annual U.S. health-care expenditures (an amount that totals in the trillions and does not account for lost job productivity). Not all the costs are monetary, of course. Although not all people living with chronic conditions experience lower levels of functioning, many experience dependence on others to help with daily activities.[23]

Our collective lack of fitness has been blamed in part on the basic fact that we no longer need to be active to acquire food and safe shelter. Since the 1950s, sedentary jobs in the United States have increased 83 percent. Some have also suggested that, as a society, we are less fit now because the standards of ideal fitness are unattainable. If we look at social media, television, and film, much of the inspiration to exercise is to attain a certain fit look as opposed to being fit so that we can move our bodies well into our later years. Ideas about our bodies are shaped by the movies and shows we watch, social media, and what our parents and coaches tell us about how we should look and how they describe or denigrate other people. There are intersections between gender, age, and race that shape our understandings of what it means to be a specific age. As the physical body changes over time, we come to reinterpret the ways our bodies are viewed by others and the meaning we give to our own bodies. The stories shared in this book will suggest that aging is very much in the eyes of the beholder.[24] Some of us take advantage of technological innovations and medial advancements to become the healthiest people the world has even seen, but this is contrasted with others who are living longer with more chronic conditions than was ever thought possible.

CHANGES IN THE BODY
AND IN THE IDEALIZED BODY

As infants, our survival depends on a caregiver. Within the first decade, we grow irreversibly and constantly, in line with genetic, environmental, and nutritional factors. By our mid- to late twenties, we reach our peak bone and muscle mass. At this point, we are at the optimal stage for reproduction and considered to be in our physical prime, as evidenced by decades of cinematic and media portrayals of beauty linked to this stage of young adulthood. Then, as our fertility, bone mass, and muscle mass decline, we enter middle age; if we are lucky enough to keep going, we embark on mature adulthood.

Physical change is obviously inevitable with age. Some of that change is visible: our hair grays, our skin wrinkles, and we begin to bruise more easily. But much of the change is internal. Your heart has to work harder to pump blood through your blood vessels and arteries. Your bones and muscles tend to shrink in size and density, which makes your bones more susceptible to fracture. Muscle loss can affect coordination and make it harder to maintain your balance. Our sex lives and self-esteem can change. Age-related changes to the large intestine can make constipation a more common experience. The bladder tends to become less elastic, plus the bladder and pelvic floor muscles tend to weaken, thus making it harder to empty your bladder completely and making you urinate more often. Our bodies burn calories at a slower rate, and our teeth become more vulnerable to decay and infection. Our sense of smell diminishes; our night vision worsens. Our eyes tend to become more sensitive to glare and have more difficulty focusing on things nearby. The lenses of our eyes tend to develop cataracts, resulting in clouded vision. Hearing high frequencies tends to become more difficult with age, as does hearing a conversation in a noisy room. Need I mention that the brain also undergoes changes that can have minor effects on memory and reasoning skills? Although living longer is something to celebrate, we often mourn the vitality of our youthful bodies.

Women face particular challenges because of menopause and navigating aging and bodily changes. Feminist scholars have highlighted and critiqued social expectations that women perform body work to retain youthful bodies that live up to ideals of bodily perfection. Women are more likely to feel the need to look younger in order to be successful at work and on the dating scene. However, men are not immune to pressures to look and perform in the perpetual state of an elite athlete. While physical attractiveness tends to top the charts of traits that society values most for women, men have long been pinned to titles like "strong" and "tough," facing pressures to look and act in ways that show no signs of weakness.[25]

However, being thin or having a physique that merely framed the bones was considered less appealing at many points in history, which was particularly true in times of famine. Even a physique that accentuated muscles was considered less than ideal throughout much of history. For the four hundred years leading up to 1900, slimness connoted poverty, old age, and the weakness of disease. Statues of goddesses from India have celebrated a full body throughout history. Look to the baroque vision of big beauties presented by Peter Paul Rubens's paintings featuring round and full-bodied women. In beautiful places like Fiji, Samoa, and Jamacia, a fuller body has long been celebrated as beautiful, while thinness is associated with sadness, poor health, and lower fertility. Men's fat clubs were all the rage in the late nineteenth and early twentieth centuries in the United States, where weigh-ins were a competitive event. William Shakespeare portrayed thinness as akin to undesirable morbidity. Among the upper classes, a full body, not slimness, was valued as a desirable quality.

Since the turn of the nineteenth century and into the twentieth century, the youthful and slim physique of classical antiquity portrayed by fit and athletic Greeks and Romans became a more mainstream ideal. With the advent of photography and film, and eventually with social media, the ideal body type featured the young and thin. Whereas celebrities in India were once praised for maintaining their full figures, Bollywood now features buff and slender stars. From the mid-twentieth century to the start of the twenty-first century, billions of dollars have been allocated to advertising and promoting a thin body.

During the cultural revolution of the 1960s, the point when many of the people featured in this book were in their twenties, new forms of embodiment proliferated. Baby boomers, those born between 1946 and 1964, experienced a distinct set of material conditions and other privileges in the postwar period that included higher standards of living, rising educational opportunities, and greater spending power among youth. The term "teenager" and a new system of age segmentation emerged with the baby boomers whereby new lifestyles were created as they entered subsequent decades, each marked by new clothes, hairstyles, music, and consumer goods. With this came the expansion of hair salons, dance studios, and specialized beauty services. Civic centers with sport and exercise facilities, such as public pools and public family fun centers, were increasingly replaced by private fitness studios that focused on individualized forms of exercise such as aerobics, weight lifting, and specific types of body workouts.

It is also important to note that, in recent decades, we have also witnessed trends that embrace different body types and stages in life. Barbie got a new body around 2000 that was supposed to appear more like a natural woman's. Plus-size and mature models and people with disabilities are now included in mainstream advertisements. Fluctuations in the ideal body type have always existed, but never have they been able to shift so rapidly. Now you can find the latest fad diet or an exercise tip for any given region of your body within seconds. At the same time, now you can and should expect to see all types of bodies represented because what it means to be fit and agile can be captured in many different types of bodies.

GET SET AND GO

This chapter started with a quote from Oscar Wilde: "Be yourself; everyone else is already taken." You cannot will yourself to be someone you are not, yet you are someone else in every moment. Aging is inevitable, inexorable change.

This book began as a quest to understand how we, as individuals and as a society, can embrace active aging by examining the stories of a remarkable set of people that were gathered over the course of roughly a decade to capture the process of aging in progress. I started this book with the hypothesis that athletes and athletic coaches would have ideal habits and would be able to provide the magic formula for staying in shape—for accessing, as closely as we can, that fountain of youth. What I have learned is that the key is in finding the best, most sustainable fitness for *your* body at every age. There are many ways that exercise habits form and fail to form. Sometimes the biggest sources of motivation come from the most unlikely sources.

I purposefully interviewed my respondents in the later stages of their lives in order to understand their perceptions of aging and how the habits they developed or failed to develop affected their mature years. Some had intense athletic backgrounds and bodies, each lives in a differently abled body, and each has struggled with numerous life challenges (including exercise). Each responded to a series of questions about their own aging process; how they took care of, abused, or embraced their bodies; their sources of motivation; how they formed healthy habits; and how they coped with life transitions and loss.[26]

Each of the following chapters focuses on a concept relevant to aging with agility and on one of a set of six generous interviewees who took the time to connect with me and share their perceptions, experiences, concerns, and advice. There is value in listening to how other people think about aging, how they come to form their health habits, and how they embrace or reject exercise and/or their own aging. Try the lessons that suit you. Then find your own approach to aging and keep practicing. Their stories may inspire you, frustrate you, motivate you, or change you—the only way to know is to get ready, get set, and go!

Chapter 2. Focus

In chapter 2, I focus on Connie, an elite gymnast who performed with the Japanese national team and spent most of her youth focused on competition, especially on winning. I include her story because once she stopped being a gymnast, she found herself lost, with no clear direction or path for her life, that is, until she focused on finding new goals for sustainably embracing her life's journey. Connie holds a set of principles about work ethics and community values that many corporate CEOs would pay good money to listen to. The oldest of the group whose stories are shared in this book, Connie still exudes athleticism and has sustained a commitment to staying fit and focused on the things that matter in life.

Chapter 3. Confidence

This chapter focuses on Janice, an incredibly confident woman, whose story is included because while she never engaged in sports as a child, she came to be in the best shape of her life in adulthood. A self-described free spirit, Janice has lived most of her life in Southern California and today is a unique combination of fiercely independent and highly constrained by youthful versions of beauty. Although her feelings about intimacy have changed over time, Janice continues to think mostly of strategies to keep moving. In chapter 3, Janice shares her aging strategies while illustrating the importance of having the confidence and good fortune to take care of yourself in the ways that feel authentic to you.

Chapter 4. Motivation

Max's life has been dedicated to hockey. He started in Canada and moved around a lot, but no matter where he went, it seemed hockey was his town's religion. After serious injury early in life, Max developed an addiction to painkillers that led to subsequent addictions. When his professional athletic career ended, Max was unsure about his identity, in constant physical pain, and in a quandary about the concept of willpower even as he tried to coach it into younger players. Chapter 4 focuses on motivation to illustrate how life as an elite athlete can paradoxically pose serious challenges to physical and mental health. Max's story illustrates that things that seem impossible can be achieved and that our later years can be our strongest.

Chapter 5. Resilience

Originally from Mexico, Yvonne moved to the United States when she was very young. In her early twenties, she became a wife and a mother and, soon thereafter, a young widow. Her early adulthood was marked by struggles to hold down work, to manage her steadily increasing body size, and to keep her footing.

In chapter 5, I focus on Yvonne to illustrate how over the course of her life, Yvonne's physical activity has become more limited and yet she resiliently persists. By mid-adulthood, Yvonne found it difficult to walk and spent much of her time seeking medical advice. By the time she was sixty, she had outlived all the more senior members of her family. Her daughter now describes Yvonne's lifestyle as neglectful and physically dependent. Although her physical activity level remains low, Yvonne takes a humorous approach to aging and maintains an upbeat personality. She is supported by her daughter, who marvels at her resilience.

Chapter 6. Optimism

Anand exercises every morning and again twice more throughout the day. Noncompetitive by nature, he has no affiliation to sports and never identified as an athlete. He is an eternal optimist, with a sense of calm and kindness that makes you want to be around him. Anand is in touch with his body's strengths and limitations. Born in India, he has lived most of his life with legs that are different in length, a consequence of childhood polio. Anand is skilled in finance and yet unimpressed by material possessions. Much of his life has been spent working numbers for various charities and working with animals. He is well read and multilingual and has lived on multiple continents. Never married, Anand lives in Berlin and enjoys a relationship best characterized by the term "living apart together" because his partner lives in a separate residence. He never wakes up wondering if he will feel motivated to move. Chapter 6 focuses on Anand because he moves as best he can, as often as he can, and hopes he will continue to do so.

Chapter 7. Commitment

Felipe was an elite judo player from Brazil and has sustained a lifelong commitment to being physically active, despite living with intense bouts of chronic pain. His body is his temple, exercise his religion. Felipe credits his personal struggles with athletic retirement, as well as his experience during the AIDS epidemic, with helping him to reestablish his sense of self-worth. He credits his competitive nature and chronic pain with launching him into personal fitness, coaching, and a sustainable pathway for aging. And he credits his long-term relationship with a younger man with motivating him to stay in shape. Now a master athlete, Felipe swims regularly, maintains his athletic identity, and works to manage his chronic pain. Chapter 7 focuses on Felipe because there is much to learn from his agile commitment to lifelong movement.

Chapter 8. Rules for the Endgame

In the final chapter, I return to the ways that contemporary social norms regarding aging influence individual perceptions of aging and individual behaviors related to exercise. From the age categories that limit our participation in a given sport to the age-related changes that slow us down, to the stopwatch that brutally imposes winners and losers, timing is everything. Societal obsession with youth and speed motivate some people to engage in fitness while repelling others. Our ability to understand how our bodies change with age, to analyze how and why we develop exercise habits, and to learn from our losses and life transitions are uniquely human. So is our ability to learn from others and adapt in order to live the best lives that we can: to age with agility. Chapter 8 concludes with advice from each of the people featured throughout the book.

2

FOCUS

Be flexible, but stick to your principles.
—Eleanor Roosevelt

A Japanese woman now well into her eighth decade, Connie is an active former elite athlete who grew up with discipline and structure. She consciously works to try new sports and exercise daily. If you could see her, you would understand that she reaps the benefits of these efforts. She is strong, fit, and agile in body and mind.

I first met Connie in Toronto through her husband's niece, Stephanie, herself a student and a competitive athlete. Both women are attractive, charming, and fiercely competitive in all aspects of life. Stephanie has an athletic scholarship and several endorsements; in Connie's day, the idea of competing in gymnastics for any reason other than the honor of the competition was unheard of, but today I would expect her to be as well sponsored as Stephanie. In fact, Connie spent most days in her childhood and adolescence focused on perfecting gymnastic routines, giving little thought to the future or a time after gymnastics.[1]

Growing up as an amateur athlete in Japan, Connie took gymnastics seriously. After representing her country at the highest levels in several international competitions, however, Connie was dismissed from the national team. She was in her early twenties, and she had fractured her wrist—for the third time—during a vault routine. This time she understood her injury meant retirement.

This wasn't like other losses. She'd lost competitions. She regularly dealt with bodily pain and injury. But she was unprepared for the feeling of disconnect and lack of focus that came with ending her career as a gymnast. Although her body was capable of doings things most people could never endure and would never attempt, Connie was worn out physically and burned out emotionally when she retired from gymnastics in the mid-1950s.

At first, it was only her stubborn wrist that seemed unable to hold itself together. Soon, however, Connie's entire body went into a state of shock (more on that in a bit). Connie would eventually find new outlets for her energy after gymnastics, and to this day she remains an athlete. I was keen to learn from a woman who exudes athleticism and has maintained a firm and consistent commitment to staying fit. Connie's life thus far demonstrates that sometimes life is full and sometimes life is lonely, but through it all, it always pays to take care of your body.

THE FOCUS WAS ALWAYS ON WINNING

Connie's early years involved multiple methods of elite training, each aiming to build focus. She remembered, for instance, how teachers at her school would place coins around the walkways, observing to see whether any student would take a coin and punishing those who did. No one inquired about *why* a student might take a coin, only that students were to learn to retain a single-minded focus on their path. When it came to physical training, Connie spoke of coaches who not only helped her train and perform but who also told her what and when to eat, where to go, and when to sleep. For well over a decade, they structured nearly every moment of Connie's young life.

As a child and teenager, Connie essentially never took a moment off. Before and after school, she trained for hours in gymnastics. Eventually she came to understand the time she spent in school and even the time she spent in competitions as her rest or break time. Her weekends were best characterized as intensive training sessions. At least during competitions there was downtime—others had to compete, after all.

While competing, whether it was a regional meet, the World Artistic Gymnastics, or the Olympic Games, Connie felt intense energy flowing through her body, every muscle exerted to its fullest potential. Over six decades later, she can still recall each way her body was scrutinized under competition and the pressures she felt to be nothing short of perfect.

> To represent your country is the biggest honor you can receive as an athlete. When you are selected to compete, it means you received best training. So you must give the best performance. I never forgot that. Every muscle fiber in my body felt the weight of that pressure. It took me decades to release that pressure. You need to find outlets for the pressure. I learned to honor my body. I learned to be patient with myself and to find ways to keep my body moving so that my mind flows in positive ways as well.

Connie's parents had no qualms about her intense training schedule. Her father was a karate master and her mother had been a dancer. They trusted Connie's coaches to guide her, and they let their only child go as far as she could push herself. They would model discipline and emphasize the importance of precise movements. Decades later, Connie recalled how her conversations with her parents tended to be about how to train more effectively, improve her routine, and minimize her food intake. Her parents expected that she would be athletic and provided a frame of reference suggesting that there wasn't anything else that she could or ought to do. Connie never questioned any of it—not even whether childhood should include time to play with friends or daydream or think about the future.

Both parents stayed physically active throughout their lives. As an adult, her mother learned to ice skate, something that can be incredibly difficult to learn later in life. Connie's parents were both highly active in various sports communities and community groups, but they were highly disconnected from Connie. To this day, Connie continues her parents' legacy of engagement with the community by becoming an active participant in numerous nationality-affiliated gymnastics organizations and community groups. She never forgot the feeling of disconnect she had from her parents, however; I could see that she still mourned her sense of isolation from them.

As is common, Connie's world as a child was small. Connie's, in fact, was uncommonly small, in part because the fertility rate in Japan was around five children per mother, and it was relatively unusual to be an only child. As well, Connie experienced the rest of the world blurred by her focus on gymnastics. But for a Japanese child, there was no hiding from World War II. It was only as Connie came of age that she began to understand the trauma endured by the society she grew up in. Traveling in early adulthood and observing how others lived helped her understand what Japan had gone through. Connie had relatives who perished in the days that followed the dropping of the atomic bomb that devastated Nagasaki. Her parents had friends who battled leukemia and those who suffered as they observed children battling with other cancers clearly related to the bombings. Connie connects the policy decisions that ended the lives of children in Hiroshima and Nagasaki with evil and regret. Today, her faith is instructive, too. She identifies with Buddhism and values how its tenets teach compassion and patience while also leaving much to be interpreted by the individual.

On a couple of occasions when we spoke during the COVID-19 pandemic, Connie reflected on World War II. In different ways, in her mind, both were points in history when the world seemed to have fallen apart, when people struggled to find their way. She repeatedly expressed sympathy for the athletes competing in the Tokyo Games whose Olympic experience and lives were being altered. Connie remembered that during and after the war, it seemed that there were so many people who had too little remorse for the devastation taking place around them. She thought about those for whom the world *didn't* fall apart, about the victors who saw others' utter ruin as their gain. She thought about how places like Hiroshima and Nagasaki were rebuilt, new families moved in, and things flourished there again.

As a child, Connie's world focused on gymnastics, and she thrived in competitions, but she insists she was never truly happy as an elite gymnast. What she did learn, she says, are good habits that contribute to her robust health today. She's competitive and adventurous, and has tried many sports, from running to tai chi, golf, tennis, gateball, swimming, climbing, sailing, surfing, and skydiving. She is introspective, reflective, and disciplined, with the motivation to keep moving every day.

PATIENCE

In addition to requiring the combination of super bodily strength, flexibility, and the ability to convince your mind to move in unthinkable ways, being an elite athlete requires that you perform under duress, often with injury, and always under intense pressure. The routines Connie regularly performed in her competitive days were stunningly dangerous, and few people could convince their bodies or minds to attempt what she did so apparently effortlessly. Who among us could hop up onto a four-inch-wide balance beam, four feet off the floor, and even *think* about performing a flip, let alone a precisely timed routine full of gravity-defying feats?

During a virtual call, when it was early morning for Connie and late at night for me, Connie came on the screen and explained that she had recently woken up and was feeling out of sorts. Sometimes, she said, the emotional pressures are harder than the physical challenges or tasks ahead of you. For six decades, she had had recurring nightmares that brought her back to a floor routine in her early years of gymnastics. She failed to stick the landing again and again, stepping just outside the allowable box on the floor. She still remembered her coaches and the pressure and the sense of impossibility: "Sometimes it is the mental that gives out. To do what we did, it requires extreme passion, dedication, focus. But this focus, it can also make you lose sight of the ways we must be to endure."

Although Connie had many competitions that she won, she still recalls her feelings of regret and disappointment each time she failed to execute her routine precisely. To hear someone in their eighties lament a loss that took place nearly six decades prior reinforces the notion that time is relative and that forgiveness is essential.

For years, Connie endured regular weigh-ins and uniform fittings. The hyperfocus on weight supposedly helped Connie's coaches track her growth and attend to safety precautions, but it felt like a burden. There were scoldings, as there often are for young elite athletes. Evidence suggests that elite athletes report lower levels of body satisfaction compared to nonathletes, likely because of the scrutiny they face. Athletes participating in sports that require weight categories or emphasize thinness also tend to have higher rates of disordered eating.[2]

As a young child, Connie knew her mother sometimes made herself throw up after a meal. Perhaps her mother had learned this during her own time as a dancer. By the time Connie was ten years old, she was regularly purging at least a few times a week. Throwing up after eating helped her maintain her weight. It also helped her maintain a sense of control over her life. By her twenties, she was throwing up nearly every day. Now she can look back and recognize that she had an eating disorder.

I had what they call bulimia. It is actually common in gymnastics. I heard someone once say, "Oh it doesn't affect Asian people." But, oh, yes, it does. Very common. Also common among us perfectionists. Maybe I was also anorexic at some points. I had all this energy, but it manifest[ed] into my being very slow. I couldn't eat sometimes, I couldn't sleep. I had a great deal going on in my head. I was upset too. I hadn't learned to be patient with myself. I didn't know myself yet.

As a gymnast, she learned to break up the "impossible" into smaller bits, each possible on its own. Like a musician learning a difficult piece, she focused on these individual portions of her routine until she was able to put the parts together. And like many elite athletes, she practiced everywhere—in her training area, in small corners of her parent's home, and she rehearsed incessantly in her mind. Once she stopped being a gymnast, Connie eventually found ways to move her body that allowed her to release energy and find joy. To this day, Connie has excellent body control.

Connie performed at the highest levels possible in her sport and moved in ways that most humans could never accomplish, yet she never celebrated her victories. For many years Connie struggled to shift her mindset from her mistakes to all the things she does so well. Now, she reminds herself to be patient and to focus on taking care of her of body so that she can keep moving. After her time as an elite athlete came to an end, she learned she could also put her life together in small pieces. She had to give herself time to just be, to discover what she was interested in and what made her happy. But before she could recalibrate, she would first crash and burn out.

THE BURNOUT

It is not surprising that someone would crash after years of intense pressure and scrutiny on their body. The wrist fracture that took Connie out of elite sports took place at her final Olympic competition. She always enjoyed the chance to compete internationally. It felt like a huge honor, and it gave her exposure to different people and cultures. But where Stephanie, her young niece, talks about going to the Olympics as if it were heaven, Connie cringes at the details of her last Olympic experience.

Burnout is often described as feeling exhausted and overwhelmed. In the academic literature, burnout is also sometimes associated with depersonalization. This is consistent with the way Connie describes the aftermath of her Olympic experience—it felt to her like she was no longer human. She was in pain. She wasn't going to be able to train anymore. She was no longer on a team. She was isolated at home with her parents. Lonely and injured, she lost the motivation to take care of herself.[3]

It took several years for Connie to go through the process of mourning the end of her time as an elite gymnast. In the first year, her body suffered the most. She gained nearly twenty pounds and watched her body transform from peak strength to one she didn't recognize. Her metabolism seemed to betray her as she struggled to find an equilibrium—as she became more independent, she could suddenly eat foods always forbidden in her competition days, and she recounted that she regularly ate rice, Spam, macaroni and cheese, and a fluffy white sponge cake that had always been off-limits. Her body reacted to the extreme change it experienced by shifting to high-energy consumption and low-energy exertion by increasing dramatically in size.

> In that first year, I lost so much muscle that my body hurt. My body shrunk and then it ballooned. I morphed into this completely different girl—woman. It was a body I didn't recognize. I didn't like it. I did my best to ignore it and then to change it.

Today her condition would likely be described as body dysmorphic disorder. Connie suffered from thinking about perceived flaws in her body. By all standards, her body was incredibly thin, flexible, and strong. But she felt so ashamed of her body that she harmed herself by throwing up regularly in order to maintain impossible standards. Connie pushed herself as a gymnast to maintain a weight that was well under what would be expected today for a person who is 5 feet, 4 inches, which is tall by today's gymnastics standards, but in Connie's day, it was considered on the short side.[4]

When her time as an elite athlete came to an end, Connie's options were limited. Women had only recently gained the right to vote in Japan, and the idea of entering a profession was not yet on Connie's radar nor her family's. At this time, it was normal for Japanese women to become housewives. Many of her peers were getting married, and Connie knew very well that she was expected to follow suit, then quickly add children. Connie had been an accomplished elite gymnast, and she wondered if there was more out there for her.

Once Connie left the world of elite gymnasts, her athletic success carried no weight, as might be the case for someone like Stephanie. There was, however, a psychic weight. It was important that Connie learn to forgive her coach for her dismissal. She had to forgive the fact that she had served her purpose on the national team, but she was deemed no longer worthy of future promise once she was no longer in her prime. She also had to forgive herself for punishing her body to the extent that she did. It took time to learn how to be patient with her body and to accept it as her home, not just a vessel for competition.

However, the time after Connie stopped competing was disastrous for her body. Connie was in constant physical and mental pain. She was also inconsistent. At times she felt slow and sluggish, unmotivated and unsure of how to structure her days, let alone the rest of her life. She was disappointed and angry. Her life was just getting started, but it felt like her world was over.

Connie had to deal with the tremendous amount of energy that she needed to burn in the wake of her athletic career. She was not offered coaching opportunities, and her parents expected her to find her way without any suggestions beyond that she ought to get married. Sometimes she felt slow and lethargic, yet she also had a nervous energy that could be addressed only by exercising. She needed to find a way to be patient with herself as she waited for her body to adapt to retirement and for the world to become a place that encouraged women to develop professional ambitions.

After she stopped training, Connie found that exercising did not help manage her weight, but it helped her keep her mind more relaxed. She repeated some of her basic gymnastic warmup exercises regularly and took up running. In retrospect, she thinks it saved her at a time when emotions were running high. She also focused on learning more about the world. Connie became an au pair and traveled, taking care of children and doing housework for families. She even worked as a cook, although she has always struggled with cooking for herself.

Connie looks at her childhood as a time when she was trained to ignore discomfort, push through pain, and dismiss signs of weakness. In her early adulthood, she tried to do the same. She recalls the constant feeling of having a stomachache and uses that sensory memory to guide her now to eat reasonable foods in reasonable portions. She once used physical discomfort to mask the emotional pain she experienced as she was cast out of the sport she grew up in and left to fend for herself.

Connie sometimes experienced intense bursts of energy; sometimes intense anger would overwhelm her, only to be followed by intense fatigue. Her memory seemed to skip and jump, turning old routines into huge errors and disastrous injuries she knew never actually took place. Connie looks back now and recognizes that, for decades, she put herself through a roller coaster of emotions over events that lasted only seconds. Now she recognizes the importance of making a conscious decision to move forward, forgive, and avoid living in the past.

> I believe the people who push the hardest burn out the quickest. This is not good. I had a dear friend on my team who hurt her head so terribly on the vault. She really never recovered. I spent years feeling anger on her behalf. She certainly can't exercise. She never really became a functioning member of society. I had such a hard time to forgive on her behalf. Nothing is worth the price she paid.

Even decades after her Olympic days, when Connie was in her mid-forties and fifties, she would walk down the street and randomly recall a judge who deducted points for a minor infraction. Other times she would be in the shower and suddenly find her wrist throbbing as her mind jumped to a coach who reprimanded her for a minor mistake. She uses this sense of injustice now to push herself to stay in shape and to motivate herself to keep moving even when she feels like being still. She has a sense of discipline that comes from painful memories of being reprimanded for minor infractions. She still visualizes her beam routine and the technical moves she performed, only to suddenly contort the memory into something absurd. She can recall intense feelings of injustice when she thinks about decisions made not only for her but also for teammates who had received deductions, punishments, or injuries that were unfair.[5]

> The Buddha said, "All life is suffering." Life can be unfair, sports certainly teaches that. It also teaches that it is important to let the mind wander because it will help you discover great times. But we must be in control of the possible paths. There are some paths to

avoid. It takes practice to learn how to avoid those paths, and it is worthwhile to learn how to do this.

The process of recovery from the pain and suffering that can coincide with a successful athletic career required Connie to focus on developing herself. Now she sometimes remembers that, in order to get stronger physically, you must endure some pain. Becoming more flexible and developing muscle both require the body to endure discomfort before improvements are gained. Connie's time as a gymnast felt like a roller coaster with ups and downs and twists and turns that often felt out of her control. The time that followed required a recalibration of Connie's understanding of her relationship to her body and her sense of her goals in life.

RECALIBRATING

In her early twenties, Connie seized an opportunity to move from Japan to California, where she worked for a family as an au pair. This experience allowed her to develop English-language skills and to see how other people lived their lives outside the world of sports. She also went to live in Australia with a family who asked her to focus on cooking. She had cleaning responsibilities and duties looking after the children, but it was the cooking that she struggled with the most. The family was patient with Connie and introduced her to another young woman working for a neighboring family who helped Connie learn about how to prepare food.

I was such a bad cook. I thought for sure they are going to figure out that I had not the first clue about how to prepare meals.

My sense of balance and my relationship to food was very off. But remember [at] that time I was still a bit chubby, so they assumed this was a sign that I was a good cook. I was also keen to get things right in the kitchen, but I was really terrible at first. Luckily the family was very forgiving. Also remember then there were also very different ways of thinking about food. Jell-O was popular!

Being in charge of the cooking for a family helped Connie learn to create new associations with food. Their eating schedule and tastes and their family style differed dramatically from Connie's own family experience. She watched the children and observed how they stopped eating when they were full and snacked when they were hungry. Her desire to be good at her job forced her into a more balanced and easygoing relationship to eating. Her experience in Australia did not cure her of all her old habits, but it forced her to focus on learning new ways of living. By the time she returned with the family to Japan, Connie had settled into a healthy weight and was amenable to looking for a husband and starting her own family.

Connie felt grounded by her experience living in the world with families different than her own, and she continued her work as an au pair when she returned to Japan. She also began trying new sports, and volleyball brought her to her future husband, Ken, who was at the time establishing himself on the administrative side of a manufacturing company. Connie jokes that her husband sees her as extremely competitive in all aspects of life. She knows that he credits her with his own professional accomplishments and laughingly says that she would have rejected him had he not worked as hard as he did: "My husband says I am extremely competitive. *Kaizen*, it means always improving or making better. I enjoy a challenge to better myself to beat a time, to win, or to do a personal best. I'm always looking to do that, to be better, not just to hang in there. That's what I strive for."

Before long, Connie and Ken married and had two sons, in sync with the fertility rate in Japan in the 1950s. As was also typical of the time, she cooked and found herself cleaning her own home multiple times a day. Perhaps a bit more uniquely, she also kept herself busy exercising at community centers or trying to find new ways to keep her body moving.

> I never thought I would have children. When I was a child, I never thought much about not being a child. I never imagined myself getting older, not until I was much older. Mid-life, then I imagined it. When I saw my mother older and declining, then I imagined it for me. Only I imagined I would just do everything differently.

Connie never imagined her life after gymnastics, so she never imagined herself to be the kind of person who had kids. Her coaches did not have children and although her own parents cared for her, they always seemed disengaged with their role as parents. Living with various families exposed Connie to ways of connecting that were warm and loving. She looked at other families and sometimes wondered what was wrong with the one she grew up in. But Connie knew her mother had suffered from neglect in her own childhood and understood that her mother lacked reasonable ways of caring for others.

> My mother died in her sleep. There was nothing wrong with her. She lived a very long life. There were times I thought she might have lived forever. It is not that I wanted her to die. It all just went on for a long time. I mean she kept on for a long, long time. She was not an involved mother or grandmother, but she had

expectations about how she was to be treated. She was unusual. She took very good care of herself, very good at looking after herself. She liked to tell me about the men who admired her. If you are the mother, you need to be aware of your audience. No one wants to hear about this! It never is perceived the way you think it will be when you talk about your bedroom life.

Connie's mother was very good at focusing on her own needs. She led Connie to gymnastics because it helped channel Connie's energy as a child and because it gave her time to do what she wanted and more freedom when Connie was training. She enjoyed the victories when Connie placed well—maybe more than Connie did—but she came to motherhood because it was expected, not because she had motherly instincts. Connie fought the idea that she would do the same. She drew inspiration regularly from neighbors, movies, and families she had observed as she developed her own way of being a mother. In time, she taught herself to focus on her children as if they were the most important things in the world and, somewhat to her surprise, they *became* the most important things in her world.

Her parents expected her to be independent as a child and young adult. But when her parents neared their final years, they each had expectations that she would focus her life on them. Connie experienced a particular resentment toward her mother for having pushed Connie so hard as an athlete and for being inconsistent with the attention she gave and the attention she demanded.

LEARNING TO SKIP

As a mother, Connie learned to monitor and moderate her competitive drive. She learned this in a very difficult way: when a friend's son died by suicide. It seemed likely that there was a connection between the pressures that Connie's friend's son faced in his adolescence and the pressures he perceived from his parents to be perfect. This motivated Connie to reconsider her relationship with her children and make a point to create opportunities in her children's lives that were different from her own.

Connie would sometimes wake up early before anyone else, just to have the quiet of the house. She would take those moments to do exercises that helped her stay limber and to meditate so that she could focus on the day ahead. Now, she wakes up and stretches; sometimes she wakes up and does cardio movements or weight-bearing exercises that help her stay limber and strong. Every day she does some exercise that helps her stay in shape. She also takes time to take stock of the stage of life her children are in, just like she did when they were young and she would assess their physical development. Now she also makes time to assess her own physical development in an adaptive and agile way.

Always mindful that they would not be children forever, Connie focused on being patient with and attentive to her children. She took them to hear music and see art museums. She still travels with them and takes them to the theater and to see movies. She has worked hard to expose her sons to sports while making it clear that she didn't expect them to become elite athletes. When it became clear that one of her sons, Masa, was an excellent runner, she worked hard to discourage her husband from pushing Masa to compete at the national level. Because she could see that they were athletically inclined, Connie pushed her two boys into several different sports. She did this with the hope that they wouldn't advance into elite levels in any one sport. By exposing them to a range of different types of art, sports, and foods, Connie has made a conscious effort to show her children, and herself, that there are many ways to find beauty in the world.

When I met Connie in Tokyo, she was keen to point out how many different opportunities there are for mature adults to exercise and engage in society. She took on the persona of a tour guide or cultural ambassador as she pointed out a neighbor who, in her nineties, had just broken the regional record at a master's swimming league event. Another friend of Connie's was nearing ninety and playing in three different team leagues. She laughed as she described people in their eighties and nineties who trained almost as much as she had when she trained with the national team in her youth.

Like many of us, Connie is full of contradictions. She is both extremely focused and driven, and incredibly flexible and open-minded. She is surrounded by people, yet plagued by loneliness. As a grandmother now, Connie understands her legacy in ways that were unperceivable at early stages in life. The idea that she might not have had children pains her. As we walked through the streets of her neighborhood in the outskirts of Tokyo, she talked about someone she knew who did not have children and another who outlived her children. There are people who think their legacy is work or in the community, but to Connie there is nothing like contributing to the world by focusing on raising another human being. And yet she also struggles because she sometimes feels very much alone in her body and in the world.

When we came back to Connie's home to have tea, she returned to the idea that being a mother is challenging but that it also helped her connect to her body and that it helped her remember the importance of practicing and being patient with her body. For example, watching her children learn to walk and especially observing them learn how to skip helped her see how difficult movement can be. As she ages and movement becomes more challenging, Connie remembers that the body is always changing, things just take a bit longer to recover from with age.

She sometimes misses her younger body, as if it were not her own body but someone else's. She laments the loss of her youthful figure, just as she laments the fact that she can no longer hug her children's toddler bodies. Yet she also notes that, as her body has changed, she has learned to adapt to new practices and to be patient. It takes time to learn to move in new ways: "It requires a great deal of patience to learn how to skip. You must really focus. I see so many of us, we are aging here, and those who do well—we focus, we practice and then we are patient with ourselves."

LISTENING CLOSELY

Connie now sees her primary role as that of listener. She enjoys many roles in her life, but she enjoys most the way that she is connected to other people. She is a mother, wife, friend, and grandmother, to name a few. Both her parents were able to model the importance of maintaining body control and agility; when it came to other aspects of life, however, such as being a person who provides protection and support, her parents did not model the ways she prefers. As her father lay on his deathbed, Connie listened as he replayed aspects of his childhood and begged for more time. She questions why each of her parents wanted to live longer lives. Each was successful in maintaining their ability to move and socialize, both factors that are often cited as important in the literature on healthy aging, but they each expressed regret that they could not live longer. Connie now believes a key component to feeling content about death is not feeling regretful about how she lived her life.

I think about my parents often. At this point, I think I have spent more time thinking about them than I actually spent time with them. They are still a mystery to me. Why they didn't value family or show that they did in the ways I would have is something I don't understand. I have many ideas about what motivated them. I am like a child still. I am still a lonely child. I have a pit in here when it comes to my parents that I cannot fill.

To Connie, legacy is not about living a long life; it is about remembering to be good to the people you care about and need to protect. She understands what it means to want to be in the limelight, to fear not leaving a legacy, to sense that you are being erased. She can still tap into that feeling of being discarded from the world she had grown up in, yet she lives her life without regret.

People who don't live their lives the way they want to regret. We must regret when we have caused harm, and there are many ways society causes individual harm. After the war, that was a different time. Things are relative; each individual, their experience is only relative to what they have been exposed to. If they don't know how much worse the world can be, how much worse a disease can be, then they react with fear. I am lucky because I could find what makes me content and because I learned how to listen. That is my role now. If I hadn't listened, I would have missed understanding what others had been through.

Connie holds on to a core set of values that guide her interactions with others while steering clear of becoming rigid or narrowly focused on a single goal. She sees how others have suffered from anxiously maintaining a narrow view of what is important to them. She even sees how she suffered in her earlier years from her exclusive focus on gymnastics.

FLEXIBLE AND PRINCIPLED

Eleanor Roosevelt's exhortation to "be flexible, but stick to your principles" is an apt summation of Connie's understanding of how to age well. The focus she held when she competed as a young woman has translated into an agile, strong, and confident woman. Connie's world fell apart in the wake of her days as an elite athlete for plenty of possible reasons. She was dealing with enormous physical pain. She had no plan for what came next. Being a gymnast had been her source of identity and connection with others for as long as she could remember. And after a single-minded focus on winning, breaking her wrist was the ultimate failure—not only did she lose her last competition, she also lost the world as she knew it.

Once she broadened her interests beyond gymnastics and the world she knew as a younger person, Connie felt happier. Her flexible mindset helped her stay physically active and positive throughout the rest of her life. In contrast to her own outlook, Connie remarked several times about people she once knew who struggled because of their extreme focus and who had since become invisible. Connie lost touch with these people who shone so brightly and then disappeared from society. She tries searching the internet for the names of competitors and athletes she admired; unless they made it to the Olympic record, it seems they never existed. Others she has seen, but their bodies have declined significantly.

> I know people, they just pushed so hard. So great and then it was over so quickly. One man, yes, he never could move without pain after his competitive years were over. When he was young, his body gave all it had. And it is a shame because he was in such

good form. I saw him about ten years, no maybe it was twenty years ago, he really could not even walk. He once, he was truly great. He could fly, he could really fly.

Connie has had the goal of aging with agility for some time. And because she is keen to age in a way that is of minimal burden to her sons and others, she has completed renovations to make her home comfortable and accessible so that she and Ken can age in place. She has handrails along the stairs, near the toilet, and in the showers. Her toilet has a built-in bidet, and her walkways are clear of any clutter. Though euthanasia is not legal where she lives, Connie is certain that she wants to take action to end her life before she becomes a "burden" to anyone else, and so she has a set of plans that would make it possible for her to terminate her life in specific circumstances should she become unable to communicate her wishes directly.

In the early days of Connie's athletic retirement, she went from being among the best in the world, representing her country at the highest levels in her sport, to feeling adrift. Now she recognizes that she went from having very little control over her life to having a life that became a completely open book. She does better when she creates goals for herself and focuses her energy on pursuing those goals. She accepts that things will never be perfect and that her body does not have to be perfect. Connie doesn't regret her instinct for perfectionism, but she acknowledges that sometimes things are out of her control. She prefers to focus on the rewards that come to those who are patient and forgiving.

Connie has lost some height in more recent decades, but she maintains a slim and muscular physique. At our most recent interview, Connie was feeling her age—and loving it. She admits that she doesn't feel as flexible and limber as she once did, but she loves moving her body. She swims almost every day and has at least four sports in her regular repertoire. She also loves doing temari, a traditional Japanese folk-art form that involves creating decorative balls with embroidery. She makes these as gifts for her grandchildren and the grandchildren of friends and neighbors, and she has also made some money selling her work.

Connie is in her eighties; her mind and body are agile. She still finds herself focusing on what she has done wrong and easily finds her mind obsessing over how to improve each task she takes on. This served her well, however, when she learned to eat in a balanced way that doesn't hurt her body. Over the years, she has stayed active and tried many sports, and she focuses on continuing to move and exercise her body. She monitors how her mind moves quickly to criticism, and she knows she can have an obsessive focus on enhancing her performance.

After Ken retired, he expressed a desire to stop work completely and suggested to Connie that they travel more of the year. However, Connie knew her husband needed to be engaged in the professional world. It wasn't just that she wanted him to continue to earn. She knew he derived a large portion of his sense of self-worth from earning and feeling that he was respected in a professional environment. She also didn't want him home all the time. Home was her domain, and having Ken around all the time would impinge on her schedule. Traveling incessantly would also impinge on Connie's regular exercise routine.

Athletic identity does not remain central to Connie's self-perception, but it is something she embraces. She believes that "athletic identity" can be ripped away when an athlete's competitive career ends but that it is also possible to continue to be an athlete if you find new goals and new ways to fuel your competitive drive. She still identifies as an athlete and as a person whose physical mobility and engagement with movement is central to who she is. She wishes there was more understanding of how we can avoid doing harm to our own bodies and to one another. Above all else, she believes that the key to a better future lies in fostering the development of individuals who focus on being flexible and patient with one another.

Connie imparts a set of key lessons that includes learning to find outlets for your energy, which might include finding unique forms of exercise or simply inviting yourself to move when the idea comes to mind. Connie finds it important to create goals and then to focus on how to achieve them. She has learned to break difficult tasks in life into chunks to practice getting better at them. She illustrates the importance of thinking about your body as your most important resource, particularly when you are a parent. Connie emphasizes the need to be a good listener at all stages in life and of moderating one's competitive drive. She does not view a long life as akin to an important life or living a long life as a personal goal. Instead, Connie focuses on acceptance and flexibility in both the body and mind.

3

CONFIDENCE

If I am not for myself, who will be for me?
—Rabbi Hillel

J anice is a woman who commands attention. She takes great care with her appearance and makes intentional eye contact when she speaks. She has excellent posture and has had a fair amount of carefully done cosmetic surgery. At our first interview, she told me, "Look, I'm quick. I love being one step ahead. I pride myself on looking younger. I'm not ashamed of saying that. Why should I be? I'm certainly not slowing anybody else down. Let me tell you, there've been many times people tell me I look younger than I am. Well, why shouldn't I? I take good care of my body. I could be a spokesperson for successfully aging."

The airbrushed poster child of "successful aging," Janice walks and moves her body easily. She is quick witted and confident. She has never considered herself an athlete or an athletic person, but she has exercised at least two hours daily for more than four decades and engages in regular treatments to enhance her body's physical strength and appearance. She loves fast cars and fast men. I knew instantly that I wanted to know, well, more.

I was first introduced to Janice at a Zumba class by a classmate who knew I would be interested in talking with her. My immediate impression was that Janice was friendly and agile. Her look is balletic. Somewhere around 5 feet, 7 inches, with a petite, refined, and sturdy frame, Janice looks graceful, strong, and delicate. She embodies a look that presupposes her commitment to exercise. She is also assertive, confident, and forthcoming.

For our first visit, Janice met me at a park in Los Angeles. One of Janice's first questions for me was to guess her age. She showed me photos of herself in her twenties, when she had wavy black hair; green, almond-shaped eyes; and a tall, thin, yet curvy figure. It was hard not to take note of the similarities and differences with her twenty-year-old self. With age, her eyes are slightly smaller, her hair has taken on a lighter shade of brown, and her face is taut and angular—otherwise, she looks nearly the same.

To say Janice is well-groomed would be the understatement of the week. She matches her shoes and purse to her scarves, she keeps her makeup flawless, and she never has a hair out of place (or allows it to gray). Her eyes *ask* you to take notice of her. And while she never regrets how much time she spends taking care of herself, Janice does not like wasting time and fills any lulls in a conversation.

Janice weighs approximately the same today as when she was in high school. Throughout her life, she never let her weight fluctuate by more than fifteen pounds. She has always painted her own toes with a range of colored nail polish as a way of regularly stretching and ensuring that she retains the ability to touch her toes with age. Her constant vigilance in exercising is like that of an elite athlete. She has many different reasons for exercising, but in many ways they all add up to doing so because exercising enhances her confidence. Exercising makes her feel steadier on her feet, keeps her from looking out of shape. Janice feels better about herself when she stays active.

Janice has always been able-bodied; her only surgeries have been for cosmetic purposes. She has some cholesterol issues and has had plenty of seasonal as well as serious but non-life-threatening illnesses, yet she has avoided major disease. Several times, Janice mentioned that when she put on a few pounds in her late fifties, she was mistaken for being pregnant. She took it as quite the compliment—akin to her pride at being denied the senior discount at the movie theater or being regarded as decades younger than the man she was dating.

For many decades, Janice worked. She had jobs in sales, as a legal assistant, and as a secretary. She married briefly (to a high-profile man she declined to discuss). Janice has identified as a divorcée for most of her life. With her divorce settlement and her own income, she purchased a condo in Los Angeles in the 1970s, at a time when many people were wrapped up in the free love movement. Janice doesn't like to dwell on her life during the hippie era, but she does like to point out that, in her day, it was much less common for a single woman to purchase property. A self-described free spirit, Janice is a unique combination of independent and self-sufficient yet highly influenced by Hollywood glamour and youthful versions of beauty.

Janice has had several longer-term relationships with men, including her four-year marriage. She has also had more than one relationship with a married man. She has several close women friends. Janice retired in her late sixties, and as she approached seventy, she realized that she had far outlived her parents and still looked considerably younger than they did in their forties. Janice is adamant that her ability to remain agile in adulthood is because she has consistently maintained a firm commitment to exercise.

THE LUCKIEST GENERATION

In 1954, *Life* magazine published an article titled "The Luckiest Generation," which described teenagers of the day as a lucky and extraordinarily confident group of kids, although they were born in the Great Depression, when birth rates were at an all-time low in the United States. This may sound surprising: the Great Depression was a difficult time, with high unemployment and low wages (for those who could find work). Many people did not have enough money to buy food, and grocery stores often didn't have enough business to stay fully stocked. For a child born in the Great Depression, also known as a member of the Silent Generation, childhood was a time to "make do without."[1]

Yet great opportunities came to this generation as the U.S. economy started to thrive again. There was less competition to get into college, get jobs, or buy first homes. This generation experienced a "double attraction" in that they were given greater opportunities to earn and so did their parents once the economy recovered. Unlike their parents, many children born in the 1930s and shortly thereafter did not have to provide financial support for their parents as they aged. A select few even inherited money when their parents passed away.[2]

Janice was born during the Great Depression to a Jewish family that was among the lucky few to flee Eastern Europe before the Nazis gained power. Her early years were spent in New York, but most of her childhood memories are grounded in Los Angeles, the city of sunshine and beautiful people. During World War II, Janice's father served overseas and her mother, like so many women, went to work outside the home in a sewing factory. Janice's childhood featured minimal adult supervision, used clothing, lots of independence, playing marbles, and occasionally going hungry at mealtime because there wasn't enough food.

As soldiers returned home to the United States after World War II, many men were eager to start families. Veterans enjoyed the benefits promised by the Servicemen's Readjustment Act of 1944 (also known as the GI Bill) including access to jobs, educational subsidies, and affordable housing. Policies were created to send women back home and out of the workforce. These policies helped bolster what's known as the baby boom—the period from 1946 to 1964 in which American women gave birth to between three and four children on average. It was a boom, indeed: during the Great Depression, the American birth rate was, on average, two children per woman of childbearing age, and today it has fallen even lower, to a level lower than replacement. We are now an aging society.

Janice's family, with five children, was somewhat larger than the average. As the middle child, she was rarely alone, even if her parents were not around much. They never locked the door to the apartment, in part because there wasn't much to steal and in part because they couldn't afford to make and keep track of keys for everyone. Although she grew up poor, Janice always had the feeling that her family was lucky. Janice rarely had new clothes or shoes, but she loved looking at magazine advertisements and watching commercials promoting the newest products. On one occasion, she received a new pair of shoes for her birthday and decided that she would save them so she could cherish their newness. The only problem was that her feet grew quickly and so she was only able to appreciate them from their box.

Growing up, Janice had neighbors who were Holocaust survivors. One of the families stands out in her memory: survivors of the Auschwitz concentration camp, they arrived with patchy hair, missing teeth, and tattoos on their left forearms. The Jewish families of the neighborhood, Janice's included, supported one another with whatever they could share, from dentistry to potluck dinners. Like other kids in the neighborhood, she and her siblings were used to not having enough, but when they met the survivors, Janice felt like she had been given a lot as a child. No one spoke to her directly about what the survivors had endured, but she understood that they had experienced things that no one should ever go through.

Plagued with the stresses of providing for five children in a country where they barely knew the language, Janice's parents were focused on making sure they could pay their rent and have food in the house. Her mother was what Janice described as "overweight and unhealthy." Shortly after she graduated from high school, Janice's father died of a heart attack. Her mother subsequently died of a heart condition within a year. All her siblings would die before they reached age seventy.

It was not until years later that she processed the toll her parents' lifestyle had on their bodies. She never observed them doing any form of exercise—in fact, the idea is laughable. In her childhood, there were no organized sports for girls to participate in, and Janice did not feel welcome to participate when her two brothers went off to play ball or sports with other boys from the neighborhood.[3] Janice came of age as the Cold War loomed and the hula hoop became a popular fad. As a young adult, Janice would come to appreciate fully how short her parents' lives were and made a point to incorporate exercise in to her own life. In her thirties, as calisthenics and jogging became popular activities, Janice was an active participant. Toward the end of the 1970s, she would shift to Jazzercise, and eventually this led into other types of aerobic activity. From an early age, Janice strove to have a long, vibrant life. However, her perceptions of what a long, vibrant life would look like were somewhat blurry.

PERCEPTIONS OF AGING

Because her parents fled Eastern Europe alone, Janice and her siblings grew up without immediate family older than her parents. As a child, she recalls having few ideas about what growing old looked like. She focused instead on media images of adults that promoted the allure of youth. With few specific examples in mind, Janice developed an affinity toward glamourized depictions of physical beauty and negative feelings about maturing. She explained, "Look, my parents died young. I had no grandparents. No aunts, no uncles. Didn't even have in-laws. Yes, neighbors—and I always had this sense that older people were sad. . . . I know it doesn't sound very nice, but I think it is fair to say I was disgusted by old people. I would see an old person in line or in a waiting room and I could just sense the decay, the smell. I would just look away."

Janice's early impressions of aging were largely shaped by the idea that nothing was more important for a woman than looking pretty and keeping in shape. Her mother spoke in tropes, telling her daughter that "boys don't make passes at girls who wear glasses" and if you go to college, it will be to get an "MRS," as in to get married, instead of a BA or BS. She told Janice and her sisters that they should focus on getting married, having children, and avoiding work. Her mother had specific ideas about how women should look and carry themselves that were very different from how she lived her own life. Janice looked at her mother's unglamorized, hectic life and knew she wanted something very different.

As is the case for many, Janice's relationship with and memories of her mother are complex. She remembers her mother as always being busy, always caring for others, always disheveled and unable to take time to take care of herself. Janice's mother held idealized versions of growing old that featured close-knit families where the mother was the center of the household, surrounded by many grandchildren. These visions never materialized for Janice's mother. When Janice thinks back on her mother's unrealized fantasies of aging, she feels disappointed and sad. Her mother's ideas about aging were very different from her own, which were largely void of children, grandchildren, or any indicators of getting old.

As a girl, Janice always understood that being pretty was important. She also understood from an early age that beauty was fleeting, which she learned from a relationship she had in her twenties with a man named Gene, who constantly compared Janice's youthful beauty to his "old wife." Gene was fifteen years older and completely taken with Janice, and he seemed to be in a loveless marriage. Janice was in college when they met at a cosmetic counter in a department store, where Janice was looking at things she wished she could buy. Gene bought a shelf full of items for her that day. During their relationship, he would even pay for her first foray into cosmetic surgery: surgery ostensibly to correct a deviated septum that wasn't really deviated. He wanted her nose to look less "ethnic" and more glamorous.

Soon thereafter, Janice became an early adopter of breast augmentation surgery. She described Gene as appealing not only because he had money. Gene, a father of two, came from a large, well-established family that owned several businesses in the area. At the time, she thought she was the only woman, besides his wife, that he was sleeping with. In retrospect, she realizes there were likely several other women in his life. She thought she would be with him forever and in some ways that brought her comfort; it also terrified her.

It's funny how time works. When I was younger, I was convinced I'd grow old with him. I was naïve and I wasted a lot of
time. . . . I finally realized [Gene] was never going to leave his
wife. It didn't happen suddenly, it's not like one day I realized
it—I was very slow, but there was a sudden turning point for me
where I looked at friends and other women who had children and
I could see what was coming in terms of how the body changes
and it terrified me.

With Gene's financial support, Janice changed her body in
ways that she thought made her more beautiful, which began a
process of erasing parts of who she was. For many years, she lived
in the liminal space afforded a mistress. She lived for Gene and
closed off opportunities to meet other men. Janice developed her
own career as she shifted from work in sales to work as a legal
assistant, but in some ways, time stood still. The years she spent
with Gene might have been years dedicated to creating a family of
her own, potentially with a man a bit closer to her own age. Janice
focused instead on erasing aspects of her identity, with a nose that
was different from the one she had been born with and a life that
was much more solitary than the one she had grown up in.

As a mistress, Janice perceived her own beauty as central
to her identity. It was what made her special and brought her
a sense of connection to the world. Men often complimented
her on her beauty. They held doors open for her and offered to
carry her bags, and they often purchased meals and groceries
for Janice. Janice felt that her youthfulness, at least in retrospect, was key to her happiness at that time. It allowed her to
live a carefree life. She would eventually try to make certain
parts, like wrinkles on her face, invisible, as if trying to replace
aspects of herself with younger versions. As she moved through
her twenties, Janice would become disillusioned with Gene.

Her perceptions of youth changed as she came to understand the importance of exercising. There was a shift when she realized that she needed to exercise to make her body look the way she wanted it to. It was a convoluted awakening after her parents' deaths and after her own recovery from breast augmentation surgery.

After her cosmetic breast surgery, Janice was in a great deal of physical pain. She had to tend to wounds across her chest and intense pain in her upper abdomen. She sometimes thought she might not make it, that the surgery would do her in. It was difficult to breathe some days and to walk. After the surgery, Janice vowed never to lose her physical strength and to make the daily effort to maintain it, to be as strong and attractive as she could be. From an early age, Janice joined the bandwagon promoting the idea of becoming older without showing the natural signs of aging. Janice sometimes spoke of aging with a sense of fear or revulsion.

> Sometimes, I don't feel like it. I get tired. I'm not a person who can sleep in, but sure—sometimes I am lazy and I skip my workouts sometimes. . . . I just know that I don't want to end up looking like my mother, ever. I have friends, they'd be so pretty if they just lost weight. They'd be really attractive if they would do a lifting class and tone up, or even just straighten up. That's motivation for you: looking at them. I have too much confidence to let things go. I refuse to end up looking like I'm an old lady. I refuse to be hunched over and dependent on someone else to help me move around. Yuck.

Today, Janice is a comparative and competitive person who holds firm to the fear of what would happen to her if she doesn't exercise. She regularly compares her weight, figure, balance, and other physical attributes with those of her friends, and she disparages the idea of letting oneself go or making no effort to alter one's appearance to be younger and prettier. She is pleased when she looks at others and deems herself in better shape than her peers.

Her daily exercise schedule is fueled by fears about what *could* happen to her body as well as by the understanding that many of her friends have started new exercise routines with great fervor, only to be sidelined by injury. Janice feels strongly that exercise is not something you can simply jump (back) into; it must be a daily, weekly, and yearly commitment.

One aspect of exercise motivation does seem to escape Janice—that it requires confidence, especially when your body doesn't look like other bodies. Our perceptions about what we think our bodies *should* look like interact with our perceptions of aging to shape the extent to which we engage in activities to keep our bodies moving. During the COVID-19 pandemic, Janice often mentioned new online exercise routines she found, a new exercise outfit she ordered, or a new piece of exercise equipment she purchased. In part, this can be traced to her sense of herself as a fit person who looks and moves better than most her age. As she puts it, "I know I'm at the age where most people are telling you how their body is falling apart. Now I'm not saying that I'm without any aches or pains, but I know more about my body now than I ever have. I know what to avoid, I know what I want, how to bring my body pleasure. I'm saying, I know what I like and I'm not afraid to explain what I don't like."

When you engage in any exercise program, you need to have the self-awareness to know why you are doing it as well as the confidence to know you are not going to hurt yourself, particularly if your body looks unique or moves in more unusual ways. Of course, having time, money, access to equipment or the space to exercise, and experience also helps. Trying to move your body the way the exercise is supposed to be executed is not always easy physically or mentally, particularly if you have a body that is never going to move the way other bodies move.

EVERYBODY BECOMES A BODY

The body is generally the first thing you notice when you meet someone. Yes, some people focus on eyes or a smile, but the overall body type is what most people take in immediately. How tall someone is, whether they seem fit, and whether they conform to our unique interpretations of desirability are factors that we tend to process at first glance.

Janice was particularly taken by Paul, a married man with whom she had a decade-long relationship. She was fond of talking about him, his body, and the ways their relationship helped motivate her to take care of her own body. Janice and Paul first met at an exercise class. Paul was handsome and tall with a sturdy build, and he was over a decade younger than Janice. There had been earlier points in her life when Janice described embracing a simple goal of finding a man with "a full set of teeth and good pills" to treat sexual impotence. She was adamant that she had no interest in becoming someone's caregiver. When she met Paul, she felt like she won the lottery. She fell in love like a schoolgirl.

The first time Janice mentioned Paul to me was in relation to a question I asked about what kept her motivated to exercise every day. Paul, she said, brought out the best version of her. She described Paul as her *bashert*, meaning a soulmate or the person you are intended to be with. Although she had been exercising regularly for many decades, she credited Paul with being a source of her inspiration to keep in shape.

Oh, probably to keep up next to him! [Paul] is gorgeous. When I'm with him, I feel desirable. You know how they say: "It's important to look your best so you can feel your best." This is the truth. With [Paul] I feel my best. Honestly, he is like a hit of coke. Do you know what I mean? You know that feeling like you can do anything. You don't need to eat; you can handle anything. Your brain literally gets rewired so you can always slide into that happy place thinking of being with him. He's my *beshert*. Yes, I think this relationship has helped me keep off the extra weight several of my friends put in our sixties. You know how it goes from the hips and thighs to the waistline.

Janice felt that all her other relationships had been preparation for her relationship with Paul. She focused on looking her best and staying slim and fit because this helped her feel more in control of her health and it helped her feel more desirable.

Janice sometimes finds herself fantasizing like an adolescent. Well into her eighties, Janice still feels strong romantic and sexual desires. Other times, Janice finds that simply being in the company of a man, sitting together, and holding hands is much more meaningful to her than any other form of interaction. While popular culture tends to ignore, oversimplify, or desexualize aging, Janice believes there is a great deal of nuance to understanding sexuality with age.[4]

AN UNCONVENTIONAL WOMAN

For much of her life, Janice has thought of herself as unconventional. She has, at various points, taken pride in identifying as a mistress, a homeowner (who does not have anyone else's name on the property deed), a secretary, and a woman without many women friends. For the most part, she also has consistently taken pride in being a woman who does not identify as a wife or mother.

Over many decades, Janice has also sought attention for her looks—from friends and strangers alike. She always keeps up with the latest fashion and is highly influenced by trends that dictate how white her teeth should look, how slim she ought to be, and how smooth her skin should look. At one point however, Janice had a reckoning. She learned from a friend that she had been referred to as a cougar, a term that refers to women in their forties or older who date significantly younger men. The term is generally understood as pejorative, an insult directed to the older woman as predatory, pathetic, and desperate. Janice took the insult as a sort of backlash for taking good care of herself and being desirable to younger men. But she also describes the pressures she felt from being the older partner in her relationship.

> There was a downside, too—probably several, I suppose. Well for me, I obsessed over every gray hair, spent a ton of money on my hair. I think it thinned because I had to dye it so often to hide the roots, you know? Not just my hair [gesturing to the top of her head], the hairs down there change, too, not sure if you know that yet! I did every treatment, tanned! Ha! I tanned! I waxed. I used every cream, injections galore. I had a facelift. Getting old is not cheap, you know. I'm saving a lot now. I showed you my moisturizers, right? Well, I had so many more.

Janice felt very invigorated by her relationship with Paul. Throughout the relationship, Janice both embraced and endured pressures to maintain a more youthful appearance. She kept constant track of where new gray hairs popped up on her body, and she studied her body from different angles to find the most youthful looking ones. Janice's relationship with Paul opened new understandings about herself, including a sense of dissatisfaction with her body's natural aging process.

> The first time he asked me to send a photo I thought, "Well, isn't this bizarre. Why would I do that?" Maybe that is what the younger gals do. Then you bet I learned how to take good pictures. But then I'd look at the photos and I'd look around on the Internet, apps, and whatnot. I saw things I didn't want to see. I realized I looked different. . . . Sometimes I had to take so many photos to get one good one for him. You know how it goes: some days are better than others. Some angles are better than others.

The proliferation of social media brought many advancements in home photography during their relationship. Janice showed me filters that could blur wrinkles and apps that add makeup to a photograph of your face. We laughed about how some of her photos ended up looking like a cartoon version of someone who might have been her significantly younger sister. She eventually mastered the art of cropping photos and altering the lighting to enhance the look she was trying to create for Paul.

Janice had to do a great deal to maintain what made her feel comfortable in her relationship with Paul. Janice pounced on any signs of her aging. Her embrace of corrective self-care practices, cosmetic procedures, and expedient lifestyle therapeutics enhanced her feelings of attractiveness. What were once understood as natural by-products of aging are now considered dysfunctions that can be fixed with prescriptions and consumer products. Her experience exemplifies a disconnect between some of the basic physiological realities that are common with age and social pressures to embrace antiaging lifestyles.[5]

BECOMING INVISIBLE

Janice is generally resistant to the concept of aging, yet she finds that there are some changes she appreciates, particularly after menopause. She appreciates how her mind has quieted as her interest in what other people think of her has diminished. She is happier in her friendships with other women, something that she did not fully appreciate until she went through menopause. Menopause, which arrived for Janice in her fifties, was a sort of shock. Always aware of her menstrual cycle to avoid getting pregnant, Janice knew something was changing right away. Menopause started with more frequent periods and major mood swings. Then she started having night sweats and endured two years of hot flashes. The transition was difficult and felt prolonged.

The physical aspects of menopause were a real blow to Janice. Her hair became thinner and grows more slowly. Gray hairs grow in all parts of her body, including her chin, the middle of her arm, moles on her chest, places where she never had noticeable hairs before. Her skin has become thinner, spotted, and creased, although she regularly uses sunscreen and gets special treatments to lighten or remove sunspots and moles.

Other changes she has used to her advantage. For example, Janice is keenly familiar with the threats of osteoporosis and knows that bone density decreases with age, so she makes sure to stretch every day. She intends to avoid getting shorter due to disc compression. Also familiar with sarcopenia, she does regular weight-bearing exercises in addition to walking regularly to maintain muscle. Always concerned about inheriting her parents' heart issues, Janice also works out regularly to help her blood pressure. Her goal has always been to be independent, and thus she exercises to ensure that she will recover quickly if she falls or becomes sick. At the same time, she has allowed herself to adopt perspectives put forward by popular culture as they relate to understandings of youthful beauty.

The transition of menopause closed off the option of being able to have children, but it opened new pathways for connecting with other women. Prior to menopause, Janice had always preferred the company of men and found women to be difficult, too busy for friendship because they were preoccupied with their own husbands or children, and less rewarding to be around. Janice enjoyed receiving attention from men and was willing to put in the effort it took to be on the receiving end of their compliments.

For Janice, menopause marked the point of no return. Not only did it solidify her status as childless, it marked a transition in the way men perceived her. She began to feel herself becoming invisible. Heads no longer turned like they used to when she walked down the street. Men who once held the door for her were now looking past her. Younger people became dismissive of her in conversations. She has to look a person in the eye to try to get their attention or at least to get them to look back at her. After menopause, Janice noticed, everyone wanted to look away. People who might have taken the time to chat with her seemingly wanted to end their interactions with her as quickly as possible. She came to experience the rejection that she had imposed on mature adults earlier in her life.

Janice attended to conventional Hollywood ideals of youthful beauty and love in several ways while holding unconventional views about marriage, family, friendship, and aging. Over the years, Janice lost several friendships with women because the female friendships could not be sustained when the women prioritized the men in their lives over their friendships with one another. Janice once had a friend who terminated their friendship because the woman grew wary of how her husband looked at Janice. Another ended her friendship with Janice because she did not approve of the fact that Janice was willing to be in a long-term relationship with a married man. Yes, Paul remained married to another woman for the duration of his relationship with Janice.

> Messages about how wrong this is are all over the place. Yes, the tabloids, the TV shows—everywhere tells you this is not a good idea. For me, I didn't feel like it was wrong. I mean, yes, I felt awful inside on many occasions. But I don't do shame. I don't feel remorse for having had relationships with a married man. I don't do regret. I don't think about this as the worst thing. In retrospect, I think the worst thing is to give up. If I let myself go and never pursued anything, that is what would have been regrettable.

For Janice, avoiding risk and not taking chances in life is most regrettable. As Janice reflected on whether she ever felt pressure to look younger because she was with a younger man, she insisted that she looked the way she wanted to look and did the things she did to alter her look for herself. Paul never asked or expected her to look younger.

FRIENDSHIP

The process of female aging is often depicted as one of loss, whereby women are desexualized and demoted because they are deemed no longer worthy of a gaze and lose cultural significance. Much has also been written about the *advantages* of no longer feeling the pressures to conform to Western ideals about youthful beauty. Some women find menopause to be a welcome transition that unveils new interests and absolves them of unwanted male attention. Janice is not one of those women.[6] Janice commented, "Hell no! Is it better to be invisible? No. Look, I understand some women might feel that way. Nah, I've never been one to get upset if a man gives me attention."

As a woman who tended to prefer the company of men, Janice was somewhat surprised by the ways that going through menopause became an opportunity to connect with other women. She described the transition as a sort of trade-off whereby there are some physical losses but also major gains, particularly in terms of potential relationships with other women. As she went through menopause, Janice reconnected with several women friends she had made in high school and loosely kept in touch with over the years. She also made some new friends that coincided with a change in occupation as she shifted from a legal assistant to secretary.

I had the opportunity to meet a friend of Janice's, Tina, at one of our interviews. In our meeting at Janice's condo in Los Angeles, it was clear that Tina very much wanted to be interviewed about her own story. Janice had described Tina as "a bit dramatic, a bit desperate, a bit pathetic. When we first met, she was an exciting new friend to me, and you know how it is—something has to click to get your foot in the door with new friendships."

Although Janice was often critical of Tina, she also adored her friend. Tina was exciting to Janice because Tina often told dramatic stories about her love life, with greater detail than even Janice would use. Tina had become a widow about a year before she and Janice met, and since then, Tina's love life has been in high gear. In addition, what fascinates Janice about Tina is a newfound interest in religion. Janice takes comfort in Tina's discovery that religion ought to be present in one's life. Sometimes Janice is critical of the fact that Tina has adopted religion only since her husband died. Other times Janice applauds Tina's interest in analyzing ways that religion helps them make better sense of their lives, particularly as they approach their later years.

> She must drive her family crazy making them go to mass all the time now. Repent, repent. I think she also uses the mass to force her family to be around her. She's not that easy to be around, you know. It's convenient though, right—we're bored to go to services as young people, yet as we age and we get closer to the judgment day or whatever you want to call it, it's comforting to have something to hold on to. Don't get me wrong, [Tina] is great but she's a taker. Don't get me wrong, we click, but at the end of the day *everything* is about her.

Janice adored Tina for being relatable and fun. She was drawn to a friendship with Tina because it presented a new connection with someone who could help Janice see the world in new ways and also appreciate her own place in the world. In conversations, Tina often brings things back to her own situation. If Janice was talking about her parents, Tina would inevitability focus on her own parents. If Janice was wearing a new ring, Tina would talk about her ring collection. Janice sees what could best be referred to as Tina's self-focus, but she also recognizes aspects of herself that might be selfish or self-absorbed. Her relationship with Tina motivates Janice to reach out to her own nieces and nephews. Tina helps Janice reflect on the type of person Janice wants to be. Sometimes Tina models behaviors that Janice wanted to avoid; sometimes Tina is great company. After menopause, Janice was ready for company that was not focused exclusively on the man in her life.

Throughout her life, Janice has had a history of erasing people. At the end of each relationship, she would close a chapter in her life, never to reestablish intimacy. Even if she would go on to repeat past mistakes, she would never go back to old relationships with a true sense of connection. Perhaps Tina represented an opportunity for friendship at a point when Janice needed a type of companionship that would not end once physical intimacy dissolved. Their friendship has lasted nearly thirty years, significantly longer than her relationship with Paul, and Janice views it as a major benefit of having gone through menopause.

Not one for regret, Janice never lamented her relationship with Paul or its end. It would be impossible for me to know with certainty why her relationship with Paul ended, but based on her descriptions, it seemed to be a combination of his interest in focusing on his wife and Janice's dissolving interest in him. When the relationship ended, Janice would get upset at herself for not waking up with the energy she once had. She spent some time mourning the loss of the relationship and took a break from her exercise routine. But she knew that exercise helped her feel more energetic and that two weeks without exercise is enough for the body to reconstitute in ways that she very well might regret.

STRATEGIC AGING

Janice described herself as someone who was successfully aging. John Rowe and Robert Kahn developed a model of successful aging that took a biomedical approach to describing the avoidance of disease and disability.[7] The term has been embraced as an optimistic way of measuring life satisfaction, even a challenge against ageist assumptions that our later years are inevitably marked by decline. It has also been heavily criticized for many reasons, including for insinuating that successful aging ought to be an outcome or binary achievement. By the original model, those of us who live with ailments, illness, disability, and limited physical or cognitive functioning, and those who fail to maintain an active or engaged lifestyle are, by definition, *not* aging successfully.

Early successful aging models were also criticized for suggesting that people have full agency when it comes to how their bodies age and how their minds change over time. In other words, early models of successful aging advocated for the avoidance of disease and disability. Failing to demonstrate successful aging constituted a personal failure. Notable gerontologists have pointed out that life experiences, lifestyles, and later life situations are shaped by a range of interconnected social inequities and factors, including racial and gender disparities, economic opportunities that differ by class, and family structures, to name a few. Like Janice, many of us are living our best lives, even if we don't look like poster children for successful aging.[8]

Janice prides herself on aging successfully in much the way that Rowe and Kahn originally had in mind. She avoids illness, she's able-bodied, and she enjoys looking and feeling youthful. But it is perhaps better to say that Janice is *strategically* aging. And if we want to be strategic about aging successfully, it turns out there are several ways to measure age. While your *chronological age* tells how long you've been alive, as I said in the introduction, it tells you very little beyond when your next birthday is going to occur.

Another measure is *functional age*. This metric is based on functional capabilities indexed by age-normed standards, and it aims to combine physiological, psychological, and social age.

The functional age of a child, for example, is assessed in terms of developmental milestones. In gerontology, functional age refers to functional capacity and can be thought of as an age that reflects your well-being and how your body functions and performs relative to your chronological age.

Your *biological age*, or how much time you have left, is not straightforward to measure, but it can be estimated based on medical tests that look at your DNA and at part of your chromosomes called telomeres. Your biological age can be altered because it is influenced by factors like whether you smoke; your diet, stress levels, and sleep quality; as well as whether and how much you exercise.

Another measure is *subjective age*, which is how old you feel. Unlike chronological age, where there is an unmovable answer, or biological age, where you need a lab to measure the results, subjective age is something you can choose for yourself. When there is a gap between a person's chronological age and how old they feel, a person might look in the mirror and feel startled by what they see.[9] That's certainly true for Janice: "I still think I'm forty. At the gym, I'm talking with a forty-year-old, and I don't even realize we're not the same age until later I look in the mirror and go, 'Oh yeah, that's right. I guess I am a little older than her.'"

There are many reasons people feel a disconnect between their chronological age and the age they perceive themselves to be, a concept also known as age dysmorphia. It's common to assume that, with age, you should feel more competent. For many people, however, reaching a position of authority, like becoming a parent or taking on a job with significant responsibilities, only makes them feel *less* competent. That is, they feel younger! The reality is that, the more competence and experience you gain, the more you realize that you know very little.

Another reason people tend to feel a disconnect between their chronological and subjective age is because they have not seen accurate representations of what getting older looks like. Much of what we see in the media in terms of representations of romance and beauty are heteronormative images of people in their twenties and thirties. When we see mature adults in films and ads or on shows and in social media, they tend to be airbrushed depictions of people who would have wrinkles and gray hair if they were not airbrushed. Combine these images with the fact that many of us now live to ages much older than our parents achieved, and we have little idea what a person our age "really" looks like.

Janice approaches this dissonance with her usual aplomb. She's a big fan of telling people that she is one year older than her actual age—a strategy she adopted at age sixty-five. As she explains, it helps her brace herself for another year and get ahead of her own biases about advancing in age. When the question of her age comes up, Janice admits that her exaggeration opens up compliments as people remark on how young she looks for her age.

Janice has another age-related strategy, which is to exercise with people at least a decade younger than her. She has been member of several different gyms over the years, and today she maintains at least two memberships at a time: one is a general membership to a gym that has a pool, sauna, and specific facilities she enjoys. The other membership is more specialized. For example, her current second membership is to a women's-only yoga studio. In the past, she's been a member at studios that specialized in aerobics, Jazzercise, or Zumba. The combination allows her to maintain a baseline fitness while also keeping herself interested. "It is the rare bird who looks in shape after decades without any exercise. I think about exercising like a face scrub—you can't just put it on your face and expect that magic will happen. You need to rub it in, carefully, put on lotion afterwards. Have a regular routine for doing this. Rinse, repeat—sounds simple. Maybe you mix it up like me, keep it interesting. But you have to stick with it."

Janice is lucky to have the means to pay for different exercise classes and a body that cooperates with her when she tries to move it. Although she grew up in a time when "girls didn't exercise," she found the confidence to make exercise an important part of her life as an adult. Now she describes exercise as her strategy for keeping her body younger and as a secret weapon for maintaining her confidence over the years.

INHALE CONFIDENCE, EXHALE DOUBT

Janice's experience demonstrates numerous ways one can be physically fit in later life. It would be easy to argue that she changed her body many times and in different ways, which demonstrates a lack of confidence in herself. But Janice sees it differently: "Look, I would not do all this if I didn't have confidence in myself. I've seen it in friends, they give up, let it all go, because they lack a confidence to take care of themselves. And in turn, I do my exercise and I feel more confident. Confident I won't fall. Confident I look good. Confident I am not my mother. Confident that I won't end up dependent on anybody."

Recall that confidence is consistently rated among the qualities needed to become a top athlete. Athletes must possess an inner strength that is required to believe in themselves, to push themselves past the fear of failure, to do things others find terrifying if not impossible (just imagine diving off a ten-meter high-diving tower or going down a forty-nine-meter-tall snowboarding ramp). Janice may not see herself as an athlete, but she knows her confidence is invaluable.

Cosmetic surgery can be a way of taking control of your body to delay the impact of aging. Janice altered parts of her body as a young woman to look more like the models she saw in magazines and later to minimize the signs of aging. Overall, 85 percent of people who have cosmetic surgery are women, many of whom undergo surgery in order to appeal to men. While Janice maintained that she exercised and altered her body for many different reasons, it was clear that men and the attention she received from men also played a major role. However, Janice has had second thoughts about having had cosmetic surgery.

> What would my face look like if I hadn't had my eyes done? I regret the breasts, because it is extra work at this point, and God knows I have enough sags and lines running across my body as it is. Overall, I might be at the point where I'm not interested in having anyone new see my body anymore. I'm a bit of a mismatch all over, I know that. All I know is, and I want you to know, make sure people do this: above all, the best thing a person can do is exercise. That is something you will never regret.

Janice's body eventually outgrew the look she had been seeking most of her life. Over the years, she eventually became dissatisfied with the ways her body grew into the cosmetic procedures she had. The transformed or "plasticized body" has been described as a performative body that illustrates often temporary and fleeting notions of beauty. Forms of bodywork range from simple mechanical maintenance, like brushing or whitening your teeth, to more complex lifestyle choices that reflect personal identity, like cosmetic surgery. Janice's body-work reflects her desire for control as well as a longing to be what she no longer is. Her experience also demonstrates that it is possible to feel motivated to keep maintaining your body, even after it stops looking the way you want it to.[10]

Our perceptions of what constitutes an attractive body depend on our life experiences and the cultural norms we witness. Janice's cultural norms are tied to her life history, her race and ethnocultural background, as well as her life in Los Angeles. As we age, notions of beauty, desire, and self-worth change but they rarely disappear. When we alter our bodies through surgery to delay or minimize the natural ways our look changes with age, we change cultural perceptions of aging for everyone. This means that general expectations of what we are meant to look like in our later years will inevitably change over time.

Janice's siblings, parents, and any older relative she could think of had died at ages she has surpassed. In the ten years I have known her, Janice has embraced being fully retired, endured the end of a significant romantic relationship, and had several close friends die. She does not fear her own death, but she notes the importance of appreciating the time she has left. There are a range of activities that she enjoys—in particular, she loves going to her exercise classes nearly every day.

Again, Janice is a *strategic* ager. She does what she can to maximize her body's ability to move and physically function by exercising regularly. She maintains the confidence in herself to continue to take care of her body. This has proven to be an optimal strategy in terms of her ability to maintain her health and agility well into her eighties—to maintain a functional age much lower than her chronological age.

When I first asked Janice if I could interview her, back at that Zumba class nearly a decade ago, she told me, "If I am only for myself, who am I?" What she meant was that she agreed to be interviewed, and she would do so in order to share her experiences for the sake of helping others. The quote is adapted from

Hillel, a Jewish Rabbi who also asks: "If I am not for myself, who will be for me?" This is another way of saying, "If I don't care, who will?" Janice learned throughout her life to recognize when there were privileges in life she could enjoy or create, and she also learned not to rely heavily on others. Her story exemplifies having the confidence to take care of herself.

Janice's story also highlights the importance of finding your athleticism even if you don't grow up identifying as an athlete. It is important that Janice did not use her parents' ages at death as a marker of her own. She has outlived most members of her family, and she lives out her years with a great deal of interest in maintaining her body's functional abilities. Janice finds it helpful to avoid the mistakes or unhealthy lifestyle habits of her parents or friends and instead uses their experiences as motivation to exercise and take care of herself. She is unabashed about her own interest in sex and appearing sexually appealing. She exudes confidence and emphasizes the need to take risks in life. Above all, she insists that exercise must be practiced consistently throughout life—we only get one body, she seems to remind us, so it's worth doing all we can to optimize it.

4

MOTIVATION

It always seems impossible until it's done.

—Nelson Mandela

When Max introduced himself as the perpetual "new kid in town," I immediately formed a soft spot for this tough guy. I, too, moved around a bit as a kid, and I know that being the new kid can be a mixed bag. On the one hand, new kids can be good at reinventing themselves from the practice of starting anew. On the other, they tend to have a sense of insecurity because they don't have a lot of practice forming long-term attachments to friends or growing accustomed to a familiar home base. Sometimes they overvalue things that folks who had more consistency in their lives take for granted, like having a regular routine.

Max *is* sometimes a ball of contradictions. He has a big personality and, in his own words, an addictive one. A regular routine was one of the first things that Max and I discussed in our initial conversation. When I asked Max to tell me about how he first got into hockey and what it meant to be an athlete, he said that he was born to play hockey. His first and most consistent memories were on the ice.

Max learned to skate about as soon as he could walk. He has fond early memories of skating while the snow was falling. When he was six years old, his parents divorced and began a steady routine of constantly moving around. Much of Max's childhood was spent in Canada, near Toronto, but there were also stints to the far north and also in the United States, around Minnesota. Max would like to think these moves were prompted by a coach; Max showed tremendous skill as a hockey player, and coaches encouraged his family to move for training. It is more realistic, however, that they moved because Max's parents each had a tough time holding down a steady job and staying in one place.

> I struggled even as a kid. Really the only real structure, consistency, you know, that I had was hockey. It was the routine, practicing all the time, the thrill of the game, that's what kept me going, you know. Was a miracle I got to practice as much as I did. Really a testament to the Canadian spirit. Community, you know. I mean we were pretty much dirt poor and I was dependent on other folks to get me places because, like I said, my folks were a bit less into me than some other kids' folks. I mean looking back, I was asking a lot. Thank god hockey is a religion—that's the thing all the towns I grew up in had in common.

Max grew up poor, in a family that can best be described as neglectful. From the time he was a young man, he was on a direct path to addiction and abusive behaviors. In a sense, hockey was the religion of his youth; being part of a team kept him grounded and motivated him to take care of himself. His parents were both Protestant, yet it seemed that their real religion was hockey. Max never questioned early morning and late evening practices after a full day at school—in fact, he loved these outlets for his energies.

ATHLETIC IDENTITY

The notion of athletic identity has been described as the degree to which someone identifies with an athletic role or devotes their time and attention to sports relative to other aspects of life. Being an athlete has benefits and shortcomings. Like many things in life, athletic identity tends to change with age. The association with a particular sport becomes less important. Being able to play the sports you want to play or simply being able to move on your own can become the priority. Max once strongly identified as an athlete but now struggles with basic movement.[1]

There is a great deal to learn from participating in sports. Max often schooled me on such life lessons. Sports teach players to be disciplined and to work toward goals. Players learn to respect coaches, to communicate, to be patient with teammates, and to be patient with themselves as they improve or heal from injury. Athletes learn to block out distractions because not paying attention can mean potential injury, points lost, the disappointment of coaches and teammates, and the pain of knowing you have not performed at your personal best. Athletes learn to be resilient when things don't go according to plan. It can be hard, however, to translate these lessons to life outside sports.

To Max, being an athlete is first and foremost physical. A person no longer capable of reaching their physical goals, he figures, can no longer hold the title. Max connects the idea of being an athlete with youth and vigor, with commitment to and love of the sport, and with actively competing. To him, competition is for the young; mature adulthood is when it is your turn to share your knowledge.

Max's athletic identity was established well before he was eight years old, when he became a left defenseman. This identity was fostered as he played on youth hockey teams and furthered when he went pro in young adulthood. As he moved into the professional level at age nineteen, Max found it easy to maintain his dedication and discipline.

Professional athletes are achievement-oriented; they push toward their ultimate goal until the point that injury prevents them from pushing any harder. While he was a competitive hockey player, Max exercised because he knew that practicing would make him better and because his coaches and teammates counted on him to perform well. The notion of playing well, assisting, and scoring for his team was deeply motivating.[2]

A serious hockey injury—a clavicle fracture—led to Max being prescribed painkillers. This started him on the path that would alter his drive to take care of his body. After three years of professional hockey, a significant knee injury prompted his coach to cut him from the team, and he would never play pro again. He would go on to lose his athletic identity and his motivation. Soon he made a routine of prescription painkillers, illegal drugs, and alcohol.

Athletic identity can mean devoting your body to your sport. What you eat, how much you drink, how you move, whether you complain about an injury, even whether you have sex all depend on your relationship to your sport. For some people, being an athlete is about being athletic. It doesn't have to involve competition or even a focus on a particular sport, it's just about moving regularly. Max disagrees with this last perspective. As soon as he stopped being an athlete in his own eyes, Max began to neglect his body. What, after all, would he be exercising *for* if not for competition?

When Max's professional hockey career ended and he stopped identifying as an athlete, he felt lost, confused, and adrift. His athletic career ended at twenty-two, at a time when many young men were being traumatized by America's war in

Vietnam. Living in Canada, Max avoided the draft, but the conflict was pervasive; he speaks of his many interactions with U.S. draft dodgers who made their way north. Transitioning from having inhabited a privileged body that was once the center of attention to being in one no longer noteworthy but always painful was a tough experience for Max.

AN ATHLETE DIES TWICE

As Max reminded me, it is often said that an athlete dies twice. The first death is retirement. And much has been written about the devastating impact a forced retirement can have on individuals, particularly athletes. When he retired, Max's life as he knew it fell apart. The identity he had for as long as he could remember disappeared almost instantly. The idea of taking care of his body or maintaining the strength and agility he developed was far from his mind. Instead, Max followed a path of destruction: binge drinking, drugs, and sexual addiction. Although he lost several teeth when he played hockey, he would do more damage to his teeth in the two years following his retirement than in his entire hockey career, never mind other injuries that were to come.[3]

Having been an athlete, Max knew better than most people the great potential his body once had. The idea that being an athlete was the core of his identity had been instilled early. The idea of *not* being an athlete could only be associated with pain. As soon as his athletic career ended, he knew he would never be as good as he once was—his coaches had told him so. His early life was full of coaches telling him to stay focused on the game, to always give his all, and not to think too far beyond his next game. Reflecting on his experience, Max could see clearly that several of his coaches had problems with alcohol and were less than nurturing when it came to dealing with injury or any form of pain.

Thus, he was unprepared to deal with pain—physical, mental, or emotional—in any real way, particularly once he no longer identified as an athlete. The traits he developed as a player seemed to be detrimental to building a life outside sports. In the early days of his retirement, Max addressed his feelings of loss, pain, and loneliness with drugs and alcohol. He struggled with the idea of not being on the ice and not being monitored by his coaches, body checked by other players, disciplined by referees, and judged by fans. Creating his own schedule and following rules were difficult for Max. He lacked role models who could show him how to function outside the structured (if still often wild) world of sports. He knew how to train athletes, but he didn't know how to take care of himself in this new iteration.

The injuries that elite athletes endure can affect their capacity to engage in subsequent activity, thus casting a shadow over their interest and ability when it comes to exercise. It is rare for a high-performance athlete to end their athletic career void of any injury, but for athletes who endure life-altering injuries, exercise opportunities are often foreclosed or require major adaptation. After serious or sustained injuries, it can become impossible to continue with forms of movement that were previously mastered to the point of being taken for granted. For Max, enduring injury was part of his sport. He never questioned his injuries on the ice—until the last one.

> Fighting is a natural part of hockey. It's in the culture. I don't care what anyone else tells you, it's part of the game. . . . I never thought twice after having the wind knocked out of me. Lost all my front teeth. Obviously, this scar here is not from shaving. But when I couldn't move—I mean the injury that ended my career—that crushed me. Completely fucking did me in.

Max also suffers from erectile dysfunction, likely a side effect from his prescription medications but possibly also related to his age and past drug abuse. Sexual impotence can also be devastating, particularly because it is often associated with masculinity and self-esteem. This dysfunction was particularly problematic for Max given the way sexual performance was tied to his status as an athlete.

> Look, I'm not gonna pretend I never loved women. I fucking love fucking women. Excuse me, sorry for that. I'll try to clean it up here. But listen, I wasn't the best character, okay? I can be a jerk. I probably had more women when I played [hockey] than most men have in their lifetime. Shit, I probably had more women while I was *married* than most men have in their lifetime. And, as you know, that was a short marriage. Thing is, having been an athlete, not being able to get it up really hurts. I mean yes, physically it is draining. Mentally it hurts. But it gets at the source of who you are as a man. I'm telling you, an athlete has to perform. Performance is everything.

Performance is essential as an athlete. Without the ability to perform, coaches lose faith and careers end. For the individual, failure to perform at the level they were once accustomed to can lead to a lack of faith in their own body. This can also lead to a lack of will to take care of their own body.

WILLPOWER

Willpower is also something that can be depleted, and it's fraught with inconsistency and challenges. Having lost his athletic identity, Max experienced challenges with willpower when it came to taking care of his body.[4]

Look, I don't know why I don't exercise. I did it for the game. Now, I have no interest. I'm not chasing ladies anymore. Now, look, I wake up and I have limitations you know. Not everything moves the way it should. . . . I get lots of pains. I don't know, maybe I just don't have the willpower?

Early uses of the term "willpower" emerged in reference to moralistic concerns about substance abuse. This connotation, in the Victorian Era, was overlaid with social anxieties regarding whether those living in poverty could uphold proper moral standards. Today, with a growing interest in self-help, willpower has continued to carry these meanings but also to encapsulate an ability to keep one's body in shape.[5]

Willpower helps avoid distraction and temptation and keeps us focused on our goals. It is something we associate with self-control and discipline. The prefrontal cortex, the area of the brain just behind the forehead, is understood to control what we chose to focus on. When we decide to linger in bed instead of getting up to start an exercise routine, or vice versa, that is the prefrontal cortex at work. Willpower corresponds to motivation; people with strong motivation may have more willpower, and willpower may help us power through when motivation is low.

There are multiple types of motivation. Internal, or intrinsic, motivation comes from within; it's about doing something for the sake of bettering yourself and learning something new because it aligns with your own interests or because it's something you value or feel passionate about. Another form of motivation known as external or extrinsic motivation describes factors outside yourself that drive you to do something.

Elite athletes know better than anyone what it takes to get motivated. Being in any intensely competitive sport requires grueling hours of practice and often pushing your body, in deeply uncomfortable and even painful ways, to its limit. To be an athlete means devoting your time, energy, and heart to your sport. Elite athletes often sacrifice the development of other aspects of their lives, including alternative career development, time with family, and dating or other social activities. Giving their best to sports takes drive, devotion, and struggle.

For the rest of us, exercise is a different kind of struggle. In contrast to elite athletes, who spend nearly every waking hour practicing or playing or thinking about practicing and playing, most adults find it difficult to make regular exercise a priority. Evidence suggests that 72 percent of adults in the United States fail to attain the 150 minutes per week of aerobic exercise suggested by the Centers for Disease Control and Prevention (CDC). Rates drop further for those living outside major cities. This comes despite an even larger body of evidence that we *all* need physical activity to maintain muscle and bone strength. We need to exercise to help our cardiovascular system work more efficiently; help keep us physically mobile; and maintain our mental health, day by day, year by year.[6]

Even when we try, we can fail to be motivated. The most popular New Year's resolution is to exercise. About 40 percent of Americans make that commitment at the start of each year, but only 10 percent of those who *resolve* to move more report any success. Getting started with a new exercise routine is hard. Committing to an exercise routine is even harder. And sticking with it can feel all but impossible.

If we have enough willpower, we can continue to engage in activities, like exercise, that offer few immediate rewards (and can instead be tiring and painful). Willpower is said to help us override impulses that prevent us from achieving specific goals. We often hear about famous or highly motivated people who wake up at 5 A.M. to start intense workouts—just the start of their amazing daily accomplishments. But what is it that drives them? Why are some of us content to stay still and rest longer while others get moving?

Max is somewhat flippant about the concept of willpower. He thinks about the term often, especially in relation to his work as a coach. He understands it as useful in motivating athletes, but he also sees it as a way to blame the individual if they don't look or act the way society suggests is optimal. As a former addict, Max worries when "willpower" is presented as a finite and exhaustible trait. People who lack willpower are labeled as weak and without any self-control, even morally corrupt. But life is more complex, and decisions like whether to exercise or not are more than simple matters of will.

BUMPS IN THE ROAD

There is always some degree of luck involved in life and in an elite athlete's career. Whether and how a referee reacts, the weather or the playing conditions, and how well your team performs are all factors outside a player's control. We say that the ways a player deals with unexpected circumstances is a question of character, that getting back in the game is a question of motivation. A review of the literature on grit, passion, and perseverance toward long-term goals suggests that psychological traits play a large role in determining success in sports. Motivation and grit are intricately connected, in part because it is not enough to have potential—we must practice and train to make use of that potential.[7]

In most professional sports, and not just hockey, players are under constant pressure to perform at the top of their game, and there are many people to help them do so. If athletes are

injured, they are pressured to "power through." Max was playing a sport that, thanks to Rule 46, allows for fighting between
players.[8] Injuries are particularly likely in careers like Max's. As
he describes it, there is a culture within hockey, perhaps common
in many sports, whereby athletes are encouraged to ignore their
injuries and continuing playing no matter what. One of the ways
members of the coaching and support staff helped players like
Max continue playing was by getting them easy access to painkillers and stimulants.

While he was a professional athlete, Max lived with a teammate whose parents owned the apartment they shared. This
permitted them both to have minimal obligations and responsibilities. Both Max and his teammate kept unusual hours filled
with practices, games, and busy dating lives. They were also
racking up injuries and using medications to dull the pain and
push through.

About a month before Max retired from professional hockey,
his father died. His father didn't have a penny to his name and
was not an upstanding citizen. He struggled with alcoholism,
had a hard time finding and keeping a job, spent time in jail, and
was perpetually dating new women. When he died, his son, a
young adult, was busily adopting many of the same behaviors. It
got worse when Max stopped playing hockey.

When Max was cut from the team, his roommate's parents
agreed to let Max remain in the apartment for six months. But
once Max found himself with loads of time; constant pain from
injuries to his knees, shoulder, and upper body; and no inclina-
tion to do anything besides play hockey (something he could not
do at that point), he took to drinking and wandering the streets.
When the six months were up, Max was addicted to painkillers:
methamphetamines, sedatives, and alcohol. It was a dangerous
combination for him and those around him.

He tried reconnecting with his mother in this period, but she had four other children and little interest in Max. His relationship with his roommate soured, and he couch surfed with various former teammates. Sometimes, he connected with a draft dodger—another young man adrift—and managed to find a place to stay temporarily. Other times he would meet a woman who would let him stay over a few nights.

> Look, I never said I was a great guy. You knew that. I was a jerk, a junkie, and an addict in every sense. . . . I was powerless; nothing was ever enough. I have many character deficits and then I also had a bad combo of needs. There was this long period of time that I wasn't able to focus on much beside my next hit.

For roughly two years, Max had no real home. The turning point arrived when Max found work in construction in his mid-twenties. What started as a desire to get money to stay high turned into a connection that would help him get sober. As a construction worker, he earned a somewhat stable paycheck. For a few years, Max managed his addictions enough, with the help of Alcoholics Anonymous (AA) and Narcotics Anonymous (NA), to hold down work in construction and related jobs.[9]

But before he would find his path to sobriety, Max had a serious injury on the job that crushed his left hand and reignited several existing injuries he had sustained from hockey. Unlike the injuries that ended his hockey career, however, Max felt that it was somehow easier to endure this new one.

> When I was done pro, I was done. Yeah, I thought, "That's it, there's nothin' left. I don't care." I hit rock bottom. It was bad, bad, bad. Yeah, I had character deficits. Never thought 'bout kicking my addictions. I really never thought I would be able to do it. But

fuck, that day I crushed my hand was bad. I blacked out. Yeah um,
I just remember when I came to, the guys were around me and the
look on their faces. It was bad.

Max never thought he would see the day that he would regain
his sobriety. But he found himself in the hospital, where one
of his few visitors was a sponsor from AA who had been
assigned to support him. He calls this visitor one of the most
helpful coaches he ever had. As he saw it, being in the hospital,
under strict monitoring and with the support of this sponsor,
was his only hope of recovering from his injuries and from his
addictions.

NEGATIVE ROLE MODELS

Many of us watch a movie about a hero and feel inspired, but we
rarely take action or change our lives based on watching someone else's life play out. Stronger motivators tend to come from
consistent interactions with people, as can be the case with a role
model, mentor, or someone who demonstrates behaviors and
traits that we want. Some of the most powerful guidance can
come from negative role models—those we see making mistakes
that we vow never to emulate.

More than two years after he stopped playing hockey professionally, Max hit his second rock bottom, when he spent a month
in the hospital following his construction injury. Now there was
another career he could never regain. He describes his time in the
hospital as being filled with fear. Fear can be a great motivator.
People are likely to be inspired by positive role models who represent a desired self, but we often find powerful motivation from
negative role models who represent a feared self. Max ultimately

came to realize that his own survival mechanisms were driven by avoiding the paths of his negative role models.[10]

It is an understatement to say that Max struggled to care for his body when his professional hockey career ended. He had no interest in looking ahead to the future or anything other than his next high. It took literally losing control over several regions of his body for him to want to change his ways. His time in the hospital gave Max a chance to reflect on his upbringing—on his father, in particular. Max explored his resentments toward his father and found, in them, motivation.

> Fuck if I'm going to be like him. Yeah, that's what I decided then. Not sayin' it came to me suddenly. Yeah, I mean, I hit rock bottom twice. And when it came to me, I was like, "Fuck yeah, I am not going to do that. This is not my path." Those memories are deep so they come to me easily. That is what helps me stay on recovery. You know, remembering that I am not going to be him.

On his path to recovery, Max had to dig deep to find the motivation to overcome his addictions. His negative role models turned out to be more powerful than other potential influences in his life. After his time in the hospital, and once he had a chance to recover more fully from his construction injuries, Max spent some time working various sales jobs until he found himself back in the world of hockey. His initial roles were in sales, then in administrative work for hockey teams around North America.

Over the years, as Max found administrative work, he spent much of his time at AA or NA meetings. He would look around at people he met in meetings and note that many threw themselves into intensive exercise regimens. Later, he would meet his wife, Ali, and her obsession with exercise would exacerbate his feelings about exercise as a less-worthy endeavor when it was done for personal gain versus more social goals, as can be the case when exercise is a means of training for competitive sports.

To Max, the fitness routines of folks he met at AA and NA were more like neurotic exercise obsessions, desperate attempts to replace one addiction with another. Max took issue with people around him who became obsessively interested in exercise for what he considered to be less legitimate reasons: because they were either noncompetitive or not affiliated with a sport. To this day, Max finds the idea of making exercise a moral obligation, in the ways some of his friends from the program did, absurd and unsustainable.

> An addict will always prefer immediate gratification. The trick is tricking the mind so you think that you are immediately getting what you want. Those addicts think by exercising like crazy, that they're getting these highs. And they trick themselves into thinking they are being so great and discipline. I see through it. That would never do it for me. I don't buy into that. I mean, good on them, but doesn't last.

Max thinks of exercise for the sake of personal fitness, and not for competitive sports, as similar to the way the Keep America Beautiful campaign of the 1970s encouraged Americans to pay attention to their litter while corporations manufactured more cheap, disposable, and profitable packing than the world had ever seen. Max views the fitness industry's emphasis on willpower as a way of creating social anxiety and obsessive self-centeredness so that people pursue the promise of unrealistic (and often expensive) goals. Max found that a more powerful source of motivation to take care of his body was harnessing his negative role models.

Max credits his father with helping him be tough and helping him take on pain without hesitation when he was playing. The injuries Max sustained from his father always healed quickly, but he still remembers the sting of betrayal that he felt when his mercurial father turned on him. Now he uses the spirit of endurance he gained from his father (however negatively) and from his athletic career to help him get out of bed and keep moving, even though his body is in near-constant pain.

LIVING IN PAIN

Max long struggled with pain and with taking care of his body. It has been suggested that the body needs to learn that danger has passed for a person to change fully and be ready to live in the present. Early exposures to traumatic injury can be difficult to overcome, leading to later experiences with post-traumatic symptoms. Injuries accrued from a life spent in a tough sport—and under the care of a tough, sometimes violent parent—plagued Max daily.[11]

Bodily injury and trauma influence how we think by interrupting our previous patterns of behaviors and actions. Systematic reviews of the literature on cumulative trauma suggest strong links between trauma exposure and persistent pain conditions. That is, we ignore past experiences at our peril—by refusing to deal with our physical and psychic traumas, we lose the chance to build the resilience that will help us overcome future challenges.[12]

When he talks with young athletes, Max thinks about resilience as a concept that can be used to help convey the necessity of readjusting focus away from pain and transferring energy more productively. Reviews of studies on resilience in sports suggest that the concept has become increasingly popular since the mid-1980s. Resilience refers to the process and outcome of adapting to challenging circumstances. It is about being flexible and being able to bounce back from adversity—in this way, it shares much with agility.[13]

Bouncing back from adversity can mean many different things, including bouncing back from the end of one's athletic career. The average athlete's career is over by the time they turn thirty. The transition generally includes going from being an all-star to being told that you are no longer a welcome member of the team. It means recognizing that your body is failing, unlikely ever to recover fully its past prowess or move beyond injuries accrued through sports.

As Max approached thirty, he was ready for yet another new chapter in life. He met a woman named Ali who he described as having the best body of any women he'd ever met. (This was somewhat ironic given that Max would go on to complain about Ali's obsession with fitness.) Ali was a great distraction from his pain initially. Max was on cloud nine whenever he was around her.

Within months of meeting her, Max married Ali, and within months of being married to Ali, Max was dismayed. He describes Ali as "the type of person who is never going to ask about your day." She was self-focused, and much of her world centered around her own exercise routine. Max believes that Ali had a poor perception of her own body and used extreme exercise as a means of controlling it. But Ali's "selfish" focus left Max feeling lonely and uncared for. Less than a year into their marriage, Max's urges to visit strip clubs and watch pornography became uncontrollable. He was also acting out, in part because of his own feelings about being out of control of his own body and in part in response to what he saw as his wife's addiction to exercise. He swears that her exercise obsession drove him away.

It's hard to explain now why it was such a turnoff for me. I am a jerk, I told you that. I guess it was the way she would obsess about herself in this way that was just selfish. She never cooked or had anything to do with food. It turned into this situation where no one else mattered and the world revolved around her. It wasn't that it was boring to listen to; it was hard to live with. I developed a vision of myself as an old man and I started to want to grow old without her in that vision.

As Max started to imagine his life without Ali, he developed a desire to live out his own life independently. Say what you will about Max's character, but in his way, Max developed a sort of agility, learning what worked for him and how to take care of himself. Somewhat humorously, Max described a lesson he learned from his three years of marriage to Ali.

Three years is my max. I like to move every three years. My pro career was three fun-filled years. My marriage was three years. That was a doozy. Acted out a bunch then. Learned a bunch. Yeah, marriage is not for me.

Now, as Max approaches eighty, he often thinks about how few years he may have left. Each day he looks at the sky and, despite his pain, he has a sense of satisfaction that he never felt in earlier decades. He feels satisfied in his independence. If he is lonely, he doesn't let on. He does demur that his body could be more cooperative, yet he thanks it for serving him pretty well given the abuse, pain, and neglect he has put it through.

RECOVERY

Max encourages athletes to exercise and recognizes it as part of their essential training, but he is steadfast: there is no circumstance under which he will ever incorporate athletics into his own life again. He is never going back on the ice or into a schedule of regular, intentional physical activity. That said, he does take care of his body by taking it easy. After a massive heart attack when he was in his fifties, Max started rejecting his father's path and continued on with his independent life without Ali, and he developed a strong will to survive.

In contrast to friends who were eager to create new exercise habits after heart attacks, work less, and devote themselves further to romantic relationships, Max found himself interested in friendships and more casual relationships and in developing higher ambitions at work. After his heart attack, Max received conflicting advice about exercise. His cardiologist advised high-impact activity and a specific type of diet. A nurse who was especially kind and helpful during Max's rehabilitation after his heart attack advised him instead to be cautious about elevating his heart rate, which he took to mean that it was better not to exercise. And that was the advice he took. Max is careful about not letting things bother him too much. He is a big proponent of napping. He avoids letting things get him angry like they might have in the past, and he avoids pretty much any exercise beyond essential walking. He jokes about driving even a few blocks to avoid exertion.

Max works to maintain and manage his health in his own way. For example, he closely monitors a schedule of medications. This prompted reflection on what it meant to be a recovering addict and athlete:

Look, I spent many years bouncing between painkillers, stimulants, and sedatives, self-medicating, right? . . . Now, I'm an old man. I'm in recovery. I have a balance that works, you know, even if I can't eat that crap. Honestly, I would never have eaten [grapefruit]. . . . No seriously, the medication I take now says I can't eat that. You know, I get really low lows. I don't think you've gone there, but I have. I have bad days, rinse and repeat. Maybe I coulda turned out better, better looking, richer? Who cares now. I've outlived so many people. I never thought I'd make it this long. But I knew I was never going to be someone who gets clean, like eating grapefruit clean or exercise on the machine or whatever, ever, period. You know, like, for what would I be doing that for? I like being old. I can't believe I made it to be an old man. I'm so much happier now. I get happier with every year. Sure, I have pain now. But, I mean, I had a lot of pain at twenty-five, right? I'm so much happier now.

While there are many days Max battles his physical ailments and pain, he never takes a day for granted. Max has shooting pains in his head, down his back, and in specific regions of his legs. He can walk and he skates, but fine motor skills are a challenge—he can write and draw, but lacing up and holding a pen are difficult. Max openly wonders whether the pains that wake him in the night have gotten in the way of leading a healthier life.

Max also laments his marital infidelities; sexual addictions; physical ailments; and personal shortcomings, including his own lack of willpower. While Max has held an incredibly strong devotion to hockey and spent an enormous amount of time creating exercise routines and training regimens for others, his own adulthood has gone by without developing any personal commitment to exercise. Overall, he just feels grateful to be alive.

Max is more anecdotal evidence in a growing body of research suggesting that people get happier with age. There were and are many days when going on seemed impossible. As he has aged,

Max's perceptions about aging have become more lucid and favorable. As a child, he never imagined getting older. In early and middle adulthood, his notions about aging were less than favorable. The models of mature adults he had were negative until he came to embrace mentors from his addiction recovery programs and his own ideas about feeling grateful to age.[14]

Approximately 20 percent of adults live with chronic pain, and 30 percent of adults over age sixty-five experience persistent daily pain; nearly 50 percent of adults over sixty-five live with some form of disability.[15] Since early adulthood, Max has lived with chronic pain, and many of his physical ailments have only grown worse over the years. Although his mature adulthood cannot be characterized as a time filled with intentional physical activities to enhance his well-being, his continued drive is a testament to his ability to push through pain and find different ways of keeping engaged. His early years with sports set him back in many ways, but perhaps they also gave him the will to endure. The recovery strategy that Max set for himself features staying away from illegal addictive substances and avoiding marriage. He laughingly claims these two rules are better for his physical and mental health than any exercise routine could ever be.

When I met Max, he had been involved with hockey for over fifty years. At sixty-five, he was at the peak of his administrative career and still as intensely focused on hockey as the day he started playing. As a player, the regular routine of practicing and the excitement of the game gave him a sense of grounding and satisfaction. Hockey would always give him a sense of home. His decision not to stay in any professional position for more than three years keeps him highly motivated, energized, and agile. He is committed to working in the world of hockey and enjoys being the "new kid" each time he makes a professional move. Making new friends helps him feel young.

Over the course of many cups of coffee, Max spoke extensively about the different drills and routines he creates for his players. He doodled warmup drills on napkins and talked about ways to develop skills and enhance tactics. He loves creating routines, especially for kids who have great potential.

> They say kids love routine, right? As you know, I crave routine. I loved the fact that practice, the warmup, playing the game isn't that different from town to town. I find comfort in that. Look, I've lied. I've stolen. I've cheated just to keep up a routine. The bottom line for me is I'm just looking for comfort and having a basic, you know, a regular routine is the better way to get there.

Max is reflective about how he manages his life and appreciative to have lived as long as he has. He can keep himself on track by channeling his energy into his work and reminding himself that most people are fundamentally good. He has experienced serious injury, life on the streets, addiction, divorce, and a devastating heart attack. Over time, however, Max harnessed positive ideas about aging that set him on living in recovery mode.

> You know, I thought that JFK getting shot was the be-all end-all. It's hard to explain now—then it felt like the world as we knew it was over. That defined things for my generation, all over you know? But this [COVID-19] pandemic, this has been rough. I'm glad we've stayed connected. I appreciate this. Several of my buddies I know they took a dive in this pandemic, back into the hard [drugs]. A friend died, too. I've been in hard times also; this one will pass. The bottom line is most people are good. I like being around people and I believe most people want to be good.

After enduring serious injury after his athletic career, Max experienced lows that brought him to a place where he never imagined being a fully functional member of society. Yet he has sustained many decades of his life in recovery. Max recognizes that, with time and experience, it has become easier for him to see the good in people and to appreciate his life. In his seventies, Max's life is full of people again. There are friends and colleagues from hockey, from rehab, from recovery. In fact, Max has named his current life chapter "recovery." The world is full of triggers, he explains, and recovery requires constant maintenance. Max works every day to fight his temptations to harm his body.

THE WIDE AND BRUTAL WORLD OF SPORTS

One hypothesis I set out with as I began the interviews for this book was that elite athletes would have insights into how to sustain exercise routines well into mature adulthood. I imagined that people whose worlds have revolved around sports would be able to share the key to what it takes to continue to push a body so that it remains active and agile. And I did find that. I *also* found that the world of elite sports can be brutal, particularly because injury is very difficult to avoid and substance abuse is not uncommon. Elite athletes' interactions with coaches fundamentally influence their careers as well as their perceptions of aging. And because of the narrow focus they have early in life, elite athletes often find themselves without concrete plans for adulthood—they, too, may not know how to sustain their bodies for later adulthood.

Early in life, Max was agile and strong, capable of moving along the ice in ways that most people will never experience. To this day, Max is the perpetual "new kid in town." He sees the world as big and wide, full of opportunities for a man of his age as long as he remains agile. With each of his new beginnings, Max sees opportunities to adjust. He finds new ways to fill the void created by the end of his athletic career. He continues his ongoing recovery, broadly speaking.

Max is no longer athletic, but he is agile and his life is built around inspiring young athletes. In some ways, Max's life has been a series of beginnings. Every time he moved as a kid, he had to start over. He had to be agile in order to prove himself to new players and coaches. Although his professional athletic career brought confidence and promise, his life as an addict was dispiriting and damaging. And then he reinvented himself again. Over many years, Max struggled to find ways to relieve stress, maintain motivation, and feel the "highs" he associated with sports—and he fell into habits that were detrimental to his health. His adulthood has been marked by constant moves as he struggled to find his way. Max nonetheless rebuilt his confidence and sense of self once he found his way back into the world of sports.

In the quote that starts this chapter, Nelson Mandela states that "it always seems impossible until it's done." Max endured many phases of life that seemed impossible, and then they ended and new phases began. His time as an athlete was seemingly impossible for someone like me to imagine enduring. The physicality of being on the ice, the intense pressures to perform, and the ability to withstand the brutality that comes with playing professional hockey would be impossible for many body types to endure. His life as an addict also has elements that seem impossible to come back from. Max did not have insights to share about how elite athletes sustain exercise routines well into mature adulthood. Instead, his experience exemplified the challenges that can be associated with having a singular focus on sports early in life and how this sort of imbalance can combine with other life circumstances to hinder healthy physical activity later in life.

Elite sports require that athletes maintain a consistent focus on winning, which can make it difficult to develop life goals beyond sports. Max's injuries, substance abuse, and limited engagement in physical activity have taken their toll on his body. Max's story illustrates that having been an elite athlete opens opportunities for serious injury and abuse, and can potentially limits one's potential to remain physically fit. His story may not be one that gives us the answers when it comes to keeping fit or staying in shape, but it illustrates that things that seem impossible can be achieved. From living on the street, Max found his way back into the world of elite sports, where he helps to train and motivate other athletes.

The lessons Max imparts include finding ways to use your potential: Share your knowledge and be generous with your story. Take powerful lessons, even from negative role models. Don't be ashamed to be gritty. "Find your passion," Max tells young folks, then helps them find ways to persevere toward long-term goals. As a mature adult, Max emphasizes the importance of not getting too angry or stressed; taking time to nap, reset, and rest; and "above all, monitor your meds carefully."

Max's story illustrates that sports can impart both healthy and unhealthy habits and that the key is to find your own path, your own way to be engaged in life. He may not personally pursue exercise, yet he believes that, with time, it is possible to become stronger, even when parts of your body refuse to cooperate. And Max sees himself as stronger and more creative than his younger self. He sees himself as a man who is aging with agility.

5

RESILIENCE

*Should you shield the valleys from the windstorms, you would
never see the beauty of their canyons.*
—Elisabeth Kübler-Ross

A friend from Yvonne's church gave her my contact information, and when I initially chatted with Yvonne, I had only a vague understanding of her physical limitations. I understood quickly, however, that she enjoyed talking about her body and exercise, but it took me some time to realize that she does not exercise. Yvonne is easy to talk with, warm and talkative. She is always keen to talk about her daughter and granddaughter who live with her, and she believes they are living the American Dream. Yvonne describes herself as Mexican American. Originally from the southern tip of Mexico, at least two thousand miles from where she's ended up in Southern California, Yvonne is bilingual and enjoys watching TV in Spanish and English. She loves staying up-to-date with current news and events. She spends a good amount of time watching cooking shows, sports, and exercise shows; following U.S. politics; and keeping up with the scandals of the British royal family.

Yvonne describes herself as a person who springs back from loss and recovers easily, and she views herself as both determined and resilient:

> I'm tough. You gotta understand this, I've been through [a lot]. I never imagined I'm gonna end up like this. You see, I started with very little. So everything I have is more than I got. Every day is extra time than I thought I was gonna get. I've been hospitalized many times. Many, many times they tell me you not gonna make it. And see I'm back. I live longer than anyone in [my family], and that's something because I had a big family.

Much of her young adulthood was spent visiting doctors, and she has found herself in and out of the hospital regularly in recent years. Still, Yvonne and her daughter, Maria, describe Yvonne as determined. The goal recently has been for Yvonne to get home from the hospital; other times the goal has been to get there as quickly as possible. Sometimes the goal is simply for Yvonne to figure out how to feel like she has more energy, to get an appointment with the right doctor, or to get the right prescription. Yvonne identifies as a strong-willed person, however, and she is always determined to "get better."

AGING IS A PRIVILEGE

Being a mother, aunt, and grandmother is important to Yvonne's identity. She grew up in a large family, and she's the type to call five times in a row if that's what it takes to get a niece or nephew on the phone. Yvonne also feels that perhaps it is because she was the youngest of her siblings that she views aging as a privilege. Her own parents were born in Mexico and moved to the

United States, where they found work in the fields picking seasonal fruits and vegetables. Their goal was to create a better life for their children. They worked with crops during the day, but they struggled to put food on the table in the evenings.

Yvonne's older siblings got the first rationing of any food when they were growing up. Yvonne was always left with leftovers and hand-me-down clothes. The family's apartment was very small; she remembers it as having two rooms, one that she shared with her older sister and her maternal grandmother, the other a space curtained off from the common area, kitchen, and dining area and shared by her brothers and parents. In addition to working the fields, her parents also did shift work, and each child was responsible for doing any work they could find around the neighborhood to help support the family. Starting from the time she was eleven years old, Yvonne worked around the neighborhood, taking odd jobs to help her parents with the rent. Her parents were generally strict, despite lacking the ability to enforce punishment if the children misbehaved because they were always working or sleeping. To this day, Yvonne sees the ability to have an abundant amount of food stocked in her house as a privilege, regardless of what type of food it is.

When Yvonne met her husband, Carlos, it was love at first sight. They met on the day of Yvonne's quinceañera. She had borrowed a pink dress with white beads that accentuated all her best features. One cousin had styled her hair into a braided updo; another had loaned her jewelry to wear. Yvonne and her sister were on the way to the convenience store to pick up drinks for her party when she first encountered Carlos. Like Yvonne, Carlos's family was originally from Mexico. He was working construction on the lot next to the store. She was fifteen and he was twenty-one. Once their paths crossed, there was no turning back.

Yvonne fell head over heels in love with Carlos, who had a handsome face and a small birthmark on his left cheek. Once he was in her life, she could think of nothing besides starting a family with him. It was difficult convincing her parents that making a life with Carlos was what was best, but Yvonne was determined. By nineteen, Yvonne was married with a baby on the way. From the time she was a child, Yvonne had wanted to be a mother. Sometimes she regrets that she never graduated from high school, but she thinks fondly about the years she worked full-time in a local clothing shop until she had her daughter, Maria. Soon after, her son, Jorge, was born. Those years with Carlos were the best times of her life. She was on the path she wanted, she felt her body cooperating, and she was in love. Yvonne particularly remembers that she enjoyed every minute of being pregnant with each of her children. Her feet swelled, but they functioned. Her arms swelled too, but they moved easily and held her up firmly.

When Carlos died in an accident at work, they had been married only five years. The news hit Yvonne like a ton of bricks. She vowed never to be with another man and to talk with Carlos, in her head, nightly. The grieving process was not easy. Catholicism and her connections with people at her church helped her feel emotionally supported and stable. Even five decades later, however, Yvonne says: "Every night, I miss him. You hear: 'Time heals all wounds.' They say, 'The grief, it fades with time.' No, you lose somebody like that, you gonna be sad no matter what, no matter how much time goes by."

When Carlos died, she began an accelerated physical decline, and Yvonne has felt that time passes differently for her than it does for others. She is keenly aware of the date and the time each day because she keeps her phone plugged in near her bed and has the TV on most of the day. But her sense of time is different from other people's, perhaps from having few years of work expectations where she was required to check in. Or perhaps because she simply goes by the beat of her own drum.

In many ways, Yvonne's life paused when Carlos died. At the time she had her children, the fertility rate in the United States was around three children per woman of childbearing age. In Mexico, it was nearly seven. Perhaps for this reason, Yvonne always laments that she did not have more children. There has always been a vacuum or space in her mind, heart, and home where she felt those other children should be.

Once Yvonne had Maria, she never returned to the paid labor force. She never thought that she was taking a pause from work to have her children. It wasn't in her nature—nor normal for her era—to spend time thinking about whether and when she would return to the workforce. She expected Carlos to be the family's provider, by her side as they figured out each phase of life together. But when Carlos died, all her planning for the future halted. He was the one and only man for her, and his loss seemed to stop time.

LOSS

Within a few years of Carlos's passing, Yvonne started having significant trouble walking and moving around. Her breathing became labored. Walking felt onerous. Her feet hurt, and her back ached all the time, as did her stomach. Soon, Yvonne's wardrobe went from skirts and pants to large, loosely fitted dresses. The phase of life when her children were young passed slowly, yet Yvonne thinks of that time as a big blur. She was always tired and had a very hard time staying awake much of the day. Once, when Jorge was just a baby and Maria was very little, Yvonne fell asleep and Maria wandered outside the apartment. Apparently hours passed and Maria wandered the neighborhood alone at an age when most children were just learning to walk. Yvonne eventually woke up, grabbed Jorge, and rushed outside. She was lucky. Maria was within a few blocks of their apartment, being tended to by a kind stranger, a parent themselves.

Yvonne recalls with clarity that her young adulthood, when Maria and Jorge were young children, was a time in which she had several instances of getting lucky when it came to the health and safety of her children. Yvonne received some insurance money from Carlos's employer, but as a widowed mother of two, life was always a challenge. Yvonne admits to being a distracted mother, but she prides herself on having been a good mother and describes her children as "healthy and clever."

Her son Jorge was always a bit of a worry for Yvonne. She feels he would have been better off with a father figure. When Carlos died, Yvonne's brothers tried to be supportive, but their help was inconsistent and they, too, died young. When Jorge struggled, Yvonne was sure the other mothers in her neighborhood suspected it traced to his lack of supervision. By adolescence, Jorge had started what would be a lifelong drug habit. Yvonne is certain that her physical and mental health challenges in the wake of Carlos's death are partly to blame for Jorge's involvement with gangs and drugs—she couldn't always be there for him in the ways he might have needed.

Jorge felt the pressure to find a source of income on the streets. Yvonne had trouble being fully present with her children while also trying to take care of her deteriorating body. One particularly painful memory Yvonne recalls is being told by a doctor that she needed to take better care of her own health and to exercise so that she could take better care of her children.

It was hard enough losing my [husband], but also I lost his stability. The money and he was the backbone. He was my backbone. I say my prayers and then I speak to him every night. When [he] died, I lost a lot. My kids, I know they [suffered], too. I lost the sense of community, too. I remember the doctor who he said if I didn't take care of me, I was gonna lose [my children]. The other [mothers in the neighborhood] they were also not kind. Yes, some they brought food. . . . They also talked behind my back. I know this is true.

When she became a widow, Yvonne felt the loss of social standing. Her whole world caved in. While she had the "millionaire's family," the supposed happy family with one daughter and one son, she was without her husband who had been the glue that held their family together. Her world became less vibrant, less engaging, and a whole lot smaller.

To this day, Yvonne carries resentment toward divorced families, believing they took what they had for granted. In her day, divorce was not uncommon, despite the church's disapproval, but she believes that when there are children involved, parents should be able to make almost any marriage work. Unless they are "too selfish," Yvonne believes that all parents should be able to recognize that there is nothing more powerful than sharing the bond of parenting children together. Families are what keep each other strong. Without family to have your back, you cannot expect that anyone else will.

When you make a choice, who you marry, then you get a choice. You stick to that because after that you not gonna get a lot of choices. Your [children] they might have troubles; they might be with somebody you not gonna like. Is that your choice then? No. You get your choice and you work on that because after that your job is to be there for their choices and then you see they gonna be there for you. Nobody else gonna be there for you.

Yvonne credits her faith, Catholicism, for helping her get through. In contrast to the catty mothers from her children's school, the members of her church were kind and compassionate, and their assistance allowed her time to grieve and to rebuild her life.

SOMATIC THINKING

For a long time, Yvonne has struggled with her body and general health. She spends a lot of time thinking about her body. She loved her pregnant body, but since then, her body has given her trouble. She is keen to talk about her ailments. Her feet don't work properly; she cannot put any weight on them without feeling unstable. She feels itchy and has rashes in her skinfolds. She often feels dizzy, lethargic, and uninterested in moving around, so she dozes off throughout the day. Maria sometimes finds her asleep with food in one hand, the remote and her cell phone in the other, and the TV blaring.

Yvonne has high blood pressure. It has also been medically confirmed that she has a form of vertigo, including general issues with dizziness and balance, and she has had a series of ministrokes. Over the years, she has had acute short-term conditions like heart burn, colds and flus, Achilles tendinitis, and bouts of depression. Her depression seems to have the most overlap with each of the other conditions, and it affects her interest in engaging in exercise.

I know I'm supposed to [exercise]. I don't. I try but it is not, it doesn't happen for me. It was hard for me after [Carlos] died, I told you there was many things that were hard. I don't know why I'm like this. [My parents], they moved around a lot, maybe too much. All my older [relatives] they ended up in bed. I remember they just stayed in the bed when they got old. I never like to get [too hot], and I get dizzy easy. I've had bad falls. I'm not interested to fall. I hate that [feeling]. I get dizzy when I'm up quickly. I know I fall easily. I don't have as many choices as other people. I always had [bad feet]. Both my parents, and they both had heart problems, in the end that's what it was, I think the heart. I don't like the feeling of my heart beats quickly. That isn't good for me. Exercising, no, that wasn't gonna be a choice for me.

Yvonne has chosen not to exercise for many reasons. She notes, for instance, that as a young widow with two children, she had no time for it. She also has the notion that exercise is not good for her, given that her father died from a sudden heart attack, and her mother and grandparents' deaths were likely due to heart issues, too. She worries about getting her heart rate too high. Yvonne often mentions exercise shows she watches, such as *The Biggest Loser* or shows that involve makeovers and feature dramatic weight loss with at-home training programs. She enjoys these shows, but she never sees the physical activities as something she would engage in.

Yvonne adapts well to the role of patient and describes herself as most comfortable when under a doctor's care. She has held this mindset for a long time and is not interested in subscribing to the idea that there is value to bodywork or to spending time shaping her body. She looks for ways her physical ailments can be addressed through the medical community while avoiding engagement in basic intentional movement, like stretching or walking.[1]

In the general population, widowhood is generally an issue most relevant to mature women because women tend to outlive their husbands (they have a longer life expectancy than men in nearly every country around the world) and because widowed men are more likely to remarry.[2] Married people also tend to outlive widowed, divorced, or separated people or those who never marry. A rich literature suggests that marriage protects and enhances health and well-being. The thinking behind this perspective is that marriage brings greater economic protection and opportunities for social connections, and makes people more responsible and less likely to engage in risky behaviors.[3]

Thinking back to her children's teenage years, Yvonne recognizes that she found herself reliant on her children. She had them buy groceries and do the shopping and cleaning. Her focus was on the cooking. She rarely went outside her apartment, and when she did, she resorted to making sure her children were with her in case she felt unsteady as she was walking. Jorge started off being very helpful to his mother. When he developed drug problems and found his way into a gang, however, his relationship with Yvonne became—and remains—strained. Yvonne sometimes feels like she lost both of the most important men in her life.

Depression is a particularly common response to widowhood, but it is not uncommon for widows to experience a range of health issues in the years following the death of a spouse. Yvonne knew she was drained, both physically and emotionally, by the loss of her husband. She views her depression as limiting her ability to engage in the world in ways that could be described as physically active. At the same time, she has always been determined to find ways to overcome what she views as her limitations.[4] For example, Yvonne has found psychological and emotional support through her church over the years. The church helped her find a more affordable apartment right after Carlos died and helped with the rent. The church also helped Yvonne navigate the public assistance she was entitled to.

They helped her with meals for many years. Church members brought Maria and Jorge to and from school when they were little until they were old enough to take care of themselves (more or less). Yvonne also had the support of a widow's group that the church helped her connect with. There are even a few women she has kept in touch with by phone over the decades.

Most of her time has been spent in the same bedroom, nearly every hour of every day of the week. Yvonne feels a disconnect with her body and senses that she looks different on the outside from the way she feels inside. She still thinks of herself as the skinny child urged by her grandmother to eat more, although doctors have told her over and over that she needs to exercise, adopt different eating habits, and lose weight. She's aware that her sedentary lifestyle is not healthy and that other people her age are more active than she is: "I know I'm a big lady. In my head I'm a skinny girl. Of course, I [know] I'm not winning Nuestra Belleza México.[5] I'm not a mover-shaker. I don't care to be in the action."

When Yvonne and I discussed exercise and aging over the years that I have known her, she was always keen to focus on her body—whether it was specific ailments or parts of her body that were a bother or ways her body looked better in her own opinion when she was younger. Sometimes Yvonne wants to share a vivid dream, often one featuring herself in a body that is much thinner and more agile than the one she inhabits in her waking hours.

IDENTITY VERTIGO

Yvonne has medical reasons for not exercising. One doctor identified her dizziness as benign paroxysmal positional vertigo, characterized by the sudden feeling that the world is spinning around you. It can be caused by simple movements, such as getting out of bed or lifting your head to look up, and it can cause nausea and unsteadiness. One doctor tried a procedure for the vertigo that had her lay down and then quickly shift the position of her head, but the procedure was very physically involved and Yvonne's doctor found her to be too heavy to lift. He prescribed for her a set of preventive pills. When she gets an episode of dizziness, Yvonne has learned to stick to her bed.

She is persistently on the hunt for a doctor who will give her a diagnosis or label for her symptoms. Yvonne wants to feel taken care of and to have something that she can attribute her aliments to. Lately, she told me, she'd been exploring whether she might have diabetes.

> I haven't felt good for a long time. I'm not gonna pretend like I was so healthy or health conscious. I'm not like [the mothers] who are so active. I didn't play sports, that wasn't something encouraged for me. We didn't have money for that. Not like people do now.

Yvonne has several doctors—and many opinions about each doctor. She does not like doctors who seem rushed. Some are more friendly than others. She prefers when they ask about her granddaughter. She takes more seriously the doctors who prescribe her medications, and she admits that she is a person who favors the idea of a quick fix or a pill to cure her.

> I gonna be happier with a prescription. I know, too many. I know that. Yes, it's gonna get confusing sometimes [keeping track]. The idea of something I can take, that's gonna fix me, that would be nice. I know [the pills] works for me, they help me. I know it's a matter to find the right ones.

Her doctors have prescribed medications over the years to address Yvonne's blood pressure, depression, and dizziness. Although at times it gets confusing, Yvonne is generally good about keeping up with her medications. She has approximately three pills she takes in the morning and five at night. Maria helps her reload her pillbox weekly, but she says that it is really Yvonne who is most on top of her medications and actually reminds Maria to help her refill the prescriptions.

A topic that Yvonne brought up somewhat early in our conversations was whether she gets dizzy or lethargic from the medications she takes. At one point, both Yvonne and Maria were interested in whether adjustments or reductions in Yvonne's medications could help her feel better or even perhaps just less tired.

> I watched a show where they say we old people are on too many meds, and it's true I get tired. I told [Maria] this is how I am, I have different blood type, mine is to move slower, and I just gotta rest more often. Also, this is how I want it. There are medications that gonna help me. I believe in this. My [mother] she never trusted medicine and she suffered. I have [benefited] from the medicine. I not gonna suffer like that. So, we went in, a couple times we went in. They say, "No we can adjust, we gonna adjust this one, but we can't take it away the other one you gotta go back to the other doctor for that one." But we had just come from that one. So you see, I think that's how I ended up with this extra one that last time.

Yvonne's recent attempt to see whether her medications might be reduced resulted in her lowering the dose of one med but being put on another new one. In some ways, drugs are a tricky topic for Yvonne. She saw her own mother, mistrustful of Western medicine, suffer with what she thinks was an untreated heart condition, and she worries that Jorge's struggles with illegal drugs are potentially a form of self-medicating. Yvonne is a firm believer in Western medicine, however, and longs for a quick fix to her ailments.

"EXERCISE IS NOT FOR THE POOR"

As a skinny child, Yvonne thought of being older as a privileged time when you got to rest and have others take care of you. Her parents, for example, worked or took care of their own parents all the time. And shortly after her father died of a heart attack, her mother took to bed, and Yvonne's older sister became the caretaker, at least for the short year left in their mother's life. Now each of her siblings have passed, and Yvonne worries that her own time is limited.

Yvonne's identity has been constructed around dealing with challenges: losing Carlos, being a single mother, enduring health struggles. These challenges encompass and affect a wide range of physical, emotional, and other dimensions of health.

When Yvonne summons herself back to the present, she realizes that perhaps she had an unrealistic perception about aging. Two of her siblings had terminal cancer, and one of her brothers died in an accident in his fifties; however, she still questions why each of her siblings died before her.

She feels that she never really understood the importance of taking care of your body and looks at people who exercise regularly as unique. Two of her nieces, both now in their sixties, are quite athletic. But Yvonne views them both as having grown up with wealth and privilege, which, to her, explains their affinity for exercise. As she puts it, "Exercise is not for the poor."

To Yvonne, exercise is a strange concept, one that is reserved for privileged people with privileged bodies. While Maria did not have a privileged upbringing, she benefits from the love Yvonne has for her. Yvonne thinks that Maria keeps herself in good shape because there was greater financial stability as she grew up than Yvonne had as a child. Maria also has good sense. Maria was provided with experiences that make her resilient and healthy. Yvonne is proud of how Maria has turned out and feels confident that her granddaughter is destined to live the American Dream.

Yvonne is always excited to talk extensively about her daughter and granddaughter. She loves sharing the story of how they came to live together, the details of their daily activities, and the recipes they cook together. Yvonne regularly praises Maria for her help with all the household cooking and for driving to Yvonne's doctor appointments. She looks forward to the fact that her granddaughter will soon be driving but also worries about how this increases the need for Maria to find a more stable source of income.

Although she does not think of aging as easy, Yvonne views getting older as the result of luck. She is proud to have made it to her seventies and thinks everyone should be proud of how old they are, no matter their age. Yvonne never thinks of herself as younger or older than her chronological age, and she doesn't mourn her youth. Still, she very much wants her daughter and granddaughter to appreciate and take advantage of these years: "Always I tell my daughter: 'Appreciate the age you are now.' At every age, I tell her, 'Appreciate this age, look how [beautiful] you are now. Wear the pretty shoes and the skirts.' I tell her, 'Wear them now.'"

THE SANDWICH GENERATION

Maria was twenty when she became a single mother. Yvonne had a three-bedroom, rent-controlled apartment with easy freeway access, so it made sense for Maria and her new child to stay. That was sixteen years before I met Yvonne and her family.

As a young single mother, Maria's world focused on her own daughter. When Yvonne's granddaughter was young, Yvonne provided substantial emotional support for Maria. Yvonne was able to marshal resources to cover their basic financial needs, and she was happy to watch TV often with her granddaughter and teach her family recipes and tips she picked up from cooking shows. Although Yvonne has not cooked for several decades, she loves watching cooking shows. When she is in a light, upbeat mood, she jokes that watching these programs is itself a form of self-medicating. She taught her daughter some family recipes that are the staples of their family meals. Since the COVID-19 pandemic, Yvonne has taken most of her meals in bed, and Maria or her granddaughter join her in the bedroom for brunch on the weekends.

The term "sandwich generation" often refers to middle-aged people who are responsible for having to care physically, financially, and/or emotionally for both their children and aging parents. Maria fell into this situation much younger than is typical. Around the time Maria was in her mid-twenties and her daughter was starting elementary school, Yvonne started to need Maria's presence when she walked. Sometimes Maria would go out during the day only to come home and find Yvonne on the floor after a fall. The two spent a great deal of time taking Yvonne to doctor appointments, seeking a diagnosis to help explain Yvonne's situation.

At one point, when I met Yvonne at her apartment, she could walk both inside and outside the apartment slowly with a walker and with Maria's assistance. She had to take breaks often, and she found it important to pace herself and not get her heart rate up too high. She struggled to move too quickly because she gets winded easily. Around the apartment, Yvonne could usually get herself to the bathroom and to the sink to brush her teeth with a walker. Her bedroom featured her bed, a small table on each side of the bed, and a medium-sized TV at the foot of her bed. Her room was full of piles of papers, magazines, and boxes. Yvonne is not a hoarder, but she does have a hard time getting rid of items. While we were chatting, Yvonne made several requests, including that I bring her the mail from her front room, get a package from a closet, and help her move several items in her bedroom. She also had an email that she wanted me to help her respond to regarding a package she ordered and wanted refunded. I was glad to have had this in-person experience because it showed me a side of Yvonne that was less obvious from the phone.

THE QUICK FIX

Yvonne has always been eager to find a quick fix for her aliments. She is not shy to admit that for a long time she wanted to look and feel better with the help of a quick procedure or a pill. Maria has bought exercise equipment over the years and set them up in the apartment, but Yvonne never used any of it. Yvonne ignored the exercise bike and the small pedal bike to exercise her arms, eventually she also ignored the canes and the walker. Maria is careful to say that Yvonne has always known she needed to exercise; she just doesn't do it.

Another doctor, maybe it was that second [doctor], he say me, "You gotta get some moving in if you want to be around for these kids." He say, "You gonna change your habits. You gotta use it or lose it." But where could I start? I'm like that. I fantasize I can suddenly get to it. Like I'm the girl on the TV.

Yvonne had a fall early in the pandemic, this time at the toilet, and thereafter she became afraid to get up and walk. This led Maria to buy Yvonne a portable toilet, placed next to her bed. In the years since, Yvonne has lost nearly all of her already limited mobility. The portable toilet next to the bed and bed rails help keep Yvonne in place. Maria uses a wheelchair to get Yvonne to the shower (luckily adjusted to accommodate the assistive device). Both women fear a fall, but they have a system: if Yvonne falls, they call the paramedics or the fire department. Then Yvonne either gets helped back into bed or taken to the hospital, where she might get a round of antibiotics or rehydration. She's returned to Maria in better shape.

Maria is confident that Yvonne has many more years ahead of her. She just isn't sure how much longer she can continue to care for Yvonne. The physical aspects are hard, but the biggest challenge for Maria is the emotional toll. She's seeing her mother continue to decline, without a substantive explanation. Sometimes Maria fantasizes that she will magically come into generous financial support. But most of the time, Maria knows they cannot afford to pay for professional care for her mother. Maria also fears losing their rent-controlled apartment should Yvonne need to go into a care facility. She is looking into hiring a friend to care for her mom, but this has proved difficult. Without using the word "selfish," Maria has described a situation where she believes her mother has led a lifestyle of neglect and indulgence that led to complete financial and physical dependence.

At this point, Maria cannot lift Yvonne if she has a fall. On several occasions, Maria has reached out to Jorge for help. Most of the time he is unavailable, but sometimes he brings food and is helpful. Still, when he's been around and Yvonne has had a fall, even Jorge cannot get her up off the floor. In the ten years that I've known Yvonne, she estimates that she has had at least fifteen calls to the paramedics to help her get up after a fall. Usually, they arrive in a team of three, check her vitals, determine she is all right, and get her back in her bed.

At one point when I called Yvonne, Maria told me to me give her a call in the hospital. She had fallen while she was trying to get on the portable toilet next to her bed. I learned that Yvonne was in relatively good health. Her vitals were good, and her blood pressure was stable. She had a urinary tract infection and some symptoms that included feeling tired and weak. But overall, she had no serious injury or disease. She was simply in bad shape.

When I spoke with Yvonne during one of her hospital stays, she was upbeat and chatty. She described her room, the nurses, and the food they served her. Yvonne mentioned that she had been in the same hospital before, when she has had a fall and needed the paramedics to help lift her. When this happens, they take Yvonne to the hospital, and Maria gets a few days of rest. In other words, when Yvonne is in the emergency room (ER), it is a break for Maria. Maria is so tired sometimes from helping her mom that she just wants to crawl into bed and sleep all day too. Over the past decade, Yvonne estimates that she has had at least three ER stays, typically lasting about one week. She always leaves the hospital feeling appreciative for her home and more engaged than when she entered. Her identity as a patient is renewed—as is she.[6]

Despite her best efforts, Yvonne never found a solution to cure her of her aliments. Yvonne found lots of doctors, several of whom told her she need to exercise, but she never was able to stick with it. Because she never got into an exercise routine, it is impossible to say precisely how her life would have turned out differently had she followed the doctors' advice. It is also hard to know whether Yvonne might have been better aided by a more fully functioning health-care system that tended more explicitly to the physical limitations and emotional ramifications of a situation like hers rather than a model focused on identifying specific physical pathologies, acute conditions, and quick fixes.

USE IT OR LOSE IT

It is difficult to explain concisely why Yvonne has become bedridden. Perhaps she never fully recovered from the grief she experienced after her husband died. Being a young widow with two young children is incredibly difficult, stressful, and overwhelming. She has suggested that she is afraid of getting her heart rate up and having a fatal heart issue like her parents. Perhaps she is afraid of falling, and perhaps it is difficult to get motivated to exercise when she feels depressed. Or maybe she declined further because of the pandemic that shut things down and encouraged her to stay home. Perhaps her medications made her tired and created conditions that would discourage any interest in extra movement, or perhaps the fact that she never exercised or played sports as a kid made the idea of exercising as an adult unrealistic. Perhaps she is sedentary because of inertia—it is difficult to get moving after you have not been moving for a long time.[7]

Sarcopenia is the term used to describe age-related muscle loss. Starting around age thirty, humans inevitably and involuntarily begin to lose some muscle mass and strength. Starting at around age forty, our muscle mass and strength declines in a linear manner without exercise. We generally lose around 50 percent of muscle by the time we are eighty years old. Sarcopenia is a significant cause of falls and fractures in later adulthood, and its treatment is exercise, specifically resistance training and/or strength training.

At any age, the tissues in your muscles will thin and atrophy within two to three weeks if they are not put to use. With muscle loss comes loss of strength and often weight loss (particularly in cases where the atrophy is associated with malnutrition or nerve problems). However, atrophy can also be associated with weight gain in cases like Yvonne's, when a person engages in very limited physical activity.

Over the course of her life, Yvonne's physical activity has become more limited. The most extreme phase of decline in her physical functioning took place during the pandemic, when she basically stuck to her bed. During the first year of the pandemic, she eliminated nearly all independent functional mobility, and she lost most of her teeth because she failed to get out of bed to brush them. Yvonne now wears dentures and is completely dependent on her family to get around. She has no backup plan beyond the paramedics and hospital, and she has no savings for long-term care or an assisted-living facility.

FOLLOW YOUR OWN PATH

In the literature on critical gerontology, the argument has been made that old age is framed and understood primarily in terms of the body and bodily manifestations, and with a focus on bio-medical manifestations of corporeality to the exclusion of social dynamics that influence our experiences of aging. Yvonne spent much of her life focusing on a biomedical explanation, thinking about her malfunctioning body or trying to find the right com-bination of pills to help resolve her ailments. This biomedical focus has often led to perceptions of aging as something to be feared or dreaded, thus creating a detrimental image of life's later stages. Yvonne's views on aging, formed when she was younger, created the idea that aging was just the precursor to sudden death. Her instinct to find a different path led her to avoid exer-cise. To avoid getting her heart rate up too high and face a sud-den cardiac event, she preferred to seek a pill that would help her feel better. The combination of inaction and taking medications has unfortunately led to a physically inactive lifestyle that has made it difficult for Yvonne to move around in the world—even within her home.[8]

The Elisabeth Kübler-Ross quote that started this chapter is about grief. It suggests that you must experience and overcome life's low points in order to experience the beauty and joy in life. Yvonne has experienced low points. In many ways, her range of experiences has been constrained by her physical limitations. Well into her seventies, her life remains liminal, paused as she perpetually awaits the results of medical exams or potential diagnoses for her ailments. Although she has been profession-ally assessed on more than one occasion, she has never received a mental health diagnosis beyond depression. Thus, it seems that Yvonne possesses a sort of resiliency. She persists and endures, she depends on others, and her resilience allows her to keep going despite her limited physical functioning.

Yvonne never expected she would live so long. She has never stuck to an exercise plan, although she has been told throughout her life that she needed to exercise to maintain her health. Getting in shape has been both a lifelong goal and struggle. At this point, she is happy to be alive—it was, she figured, her duty to keep going for her family—and not particularly keen on changing her routine.

The takeways she imparts include learning to take pride in what you've endured. The self-perception that you are a determined person can help create resilience. She also stresses being gentle when dealing with loss, learning to cope, and finding supports like the church or neighbors to help. If Yvonne's story leaves you worried for Maria, that is understandable. Maria's story is still unfolding, but it is clear that she may be just as resilient as her mother, in no small part because of her insistence that she will not follow her mother's path.

As Yvonne approaches eighty, she has outlived her siblings. The burden of her limited movement will most likely be borne by Maria and by the health-care system, both of which Yvonne trusts but neither of which can offer any solution. At one point, Maria said that if you want to live a long time, stay inside. Yvonne joins a growing group of mature adults who haven't been moving for a while but may continue living for many years. Yvonne finds joy in her family, her cooking shows, and phone calls. Maria holds things together and keeps herself physically active. While this may not be what we think of as aging with agility, the resilience of these women is a lesson in itself.

6

OPTIMISM

Start where you are. Use what you have. Do what you can.
—Arthur Ashe

Anand was born in Nagpur, India, to a young, poor, unmarried mother who was unable to raise him. Anand assumes his birth mother went on to have other children and, given that the fertility rate in India around the time he was born and for several decades after was around six children per woman, he is probably right. The fertility rate in India is currently just over two, as is the case in many parts of the world, and the proportion of mature adults in India has increased steadily for over a decade. By 2050, the country is poised to have nearly 350 million people over age sixty. This dramatic societal transformation will have far-reaching implications for India's health-care systems, families, and society at large.

Anand considers himself very lucky. The prospects for an abandoned child in India in the 1930s were not great, and his childhood was off to a rough start, that is, until a British family decided to adopt him. As the story goes, he joined two other adopted children, around the same age and from the same city.

Their adoptive father worked for the British government, and their mother was a homemaker eager for children but unable to have them biologically. Anand and his family lived in India until Anand and his siblings were around ten years old. Then they moved to a town near London.

While the family lived in India, they had a large household staff. When Anand was around five years old, his father traveled to London to plan the family's move. The rest of the family, including several members of the staff, caught polio while he was gone. Anand and two of the nannies had the worst of it: in addition to the flulike symptoms, they had severe headaches, neck pain, and stiffness. One nanny passed away, and Anand remembers being left to fend for himself (whether it was for hours or days, he does not know). Anand survived, but with several impacts on his body, one being extreme difficulty walking. To this day, his right leg is shorter than the other and other parts of his body grew in ways he describes as "out of proportion."

Throughout his childhood, more than a few doctors indicated that Anand would never walk again. One doctor even suggested that his parents commit him to an institution where he could be "better looked after"—better, even, than with the assistants at home who made sure he was "exceedingly well cared for." His parents did not institutionalize him, however, and he remained at home with his family.

His childhood was marked by a strong sense of love from his mother and a bond with his siblings, even if he always felt there were more similarities between the other two children. Anand's siblings would often run ahead of him; play while he worked with physical therapists; or take off on their bicycles while he remained in his wheelchair, close enough to know what they were doing but not able to participate. They weren't malicious; they were just kids.

Christianity was important to Anand's family. One of the family's ideals was to "love your neighbor as yourself," and thus they would buy and distribute food to people in their community. As he helped his family in this effort, Anand sometimes observed that his body was different. Sometimes, particularly when the family was distributing food in the community, he encountered people who were not so different from himself. Even if his body would never move like his siblings' bodies, Anand learned the value of getting himself around, taking care of his body, and eating well. He resolved that he would never remain still if there was a way he could muster the ability to move.

After the polio, Anand's father made him feel he was a disappointment. His brother was the favored child, perhaps because he shared their father's political views or perhaps because he was more physically capable. His sister was constantly doted on. Anand was different: "I was, am certainly disfigured, disabled. We don't call it that. Sometimes I hear 'differently abled.' Well anyway, this was simply not appealing to my father who was charitable, yes, but not if there was a semblance of reckoning someone wasn't top notch. In that case, he was—let's just say, 'dismissive.'"

To this day, Anand credits his father for helping him become someone who is mindful that being cared for can inhibit one's progress in becoming independent. Much of Anand's childhood and adolescence was spent reading and learning from whatever books he could get his hands on. Whenever he could, he had someone take him to the library to get books on history, world religions, Hinduism, and exercise. He was always keen on the last topic, motivated to find the right exercises in part because he wanted to move the way that would gain his father's approval and in part because he wanted to exert control over his sometimes inconsistent and unwilling body.

From an early age, Anand made a ritual of doing exercises every day to improve his strength based on whatever he learned from books and his visits with nurses. Sometimes he made up his own exercises. Anand simulated weights by lifting books. He did movements that would likely now be labeled "Pilates" by stretching out like a cat and tensing his stomach muscles. Much of what appeals to him now is a form of yoga that he has modified to suit his abilities and believes gives him physical and mental strength.[1]

As an adolescent, Anand embraced Hinduism; as a mature adult, he is grateful for the way it has helped him see the world, how it has provided him with a code of behavior that guides him toward kindness, balance, and self-control. Studying economics has also influenced Anand's perception of the world. He credits it with everything from helping him understand scarcity to helping him make decisions about how to spend his money wisely and how best to allocate his time. For Anand, physical and mental health are intricately linked. Exercise and movement are key to his ability to find contentment in this life.

Growing up, Anand recognized the value of taking care of his own body, even as he came to embrace Hinduism and the idea that he would not always live in this body. It is fair to say that the family Anand and his siblings grew up in had a great deal of wealth, particularly relative to the castes into which they were born.

"ONE OF THE LUCKY ONES"

Anand always considers himself "one of the lucky ones." For someone so hardworking, I have always found his understanding of luck somewhat ironic. Anand and I met in Berkeley,

California, over twenty years ago when I was an undergraduate student and he was completing a PhD in economics. Neither of us can recall exactly how we first met—perhaps at a contentious housing co-op meeting, or perhaps we bonded as I struggled with economics coursework. Of course, Anand says our meeting was "pure luck."

In those days, Anand used a manual wheelchair to get around and operated it on his own. He knew to avoid certain spots of the campus where wheelchairs could fall over easily. At the time, Anand was in his early forties—an age that many likely consider an older-than-average student. But age makes no difference to Anand. There were no precise records from his birth, he believes his birthday is a chosen one.

Most knowledgeable people, says Anand, are smart enough to know there is a great deal they don't know. By the time he became a graduate student in economics, Anand not only had a terrific foundation for understanding complex econometric principles but also had a firm grasp of many subjects, including religion, music, history, and political science. In the time before his PhD program, he had the benefit of alternating between being a scholar and working for the private equity company his father founded. He is lucky that learning comes easy to him. It is movement that is difficult.

After having grown up with staff who helped him get around, Anand feared he would require assistance for the rest of his life. However, Anand considered himself lucky in his Berkeley days because the housing he lived in included many people who required assistance for their activities of daily living (ADLs), such as eating, personal hygiene and grooming, dressing, toileting, and getting from place to place. He regularly commented on his relative bodily privilege; he took pride in the fact that he didn't have a caregiver and regularly described himself as an optimist.

Most economists would agree that luck is endogenous; good luck is a result of hard work, planning, and firm foundations. Lucky people, in this view, are those who are observant and put themselves out there. They find money on the street because they observe their surroundings; if they win the lottery it is because they plan ahead and buy the lottery ticket; they get ahead because they started in good circumstances and built on these solid foundations. Anand's idea of luck, on the other hand, is a little more like *being charmed*. To him, each milestone in his life has been the result of a lucky break.

> I always knew I was lucky. There were many other children who had it much worse. I know people look at me and think I am limited or whatnot. I know there also those who see how lucky I have been. I have never looked quite like everyone else. I am not convinced there is any value to "be like everyone else." I am loyal to my exercises, and I am not interested to deal with other people's ideas that there is one type of body [that] is supreme.

Anand is an incredibly hardworking person—and he has to be. To maintain basic, everyday movement, Anand must engage in regular stretching and specific exercises that are time-consuming and effortful. He's had the benefit of training with professional physical therapists to maximize his functional mobility, but the complex movements require discipline and motivation—a bit like learning the ins and outs of economics.

BURDENS

Some people might have felt relatively disadvantaged, yet Anand never looks at the world this way. Well into adulthood, his siblings enjoyed fancier homes, cars, and lifestyles. But Anand has a different take on life, largely manifested through his different religious ideology. For instance, at their annual Christmas gathering, when his nieces and nephews wore their finest clothes and gathered under the largest tree money could buy, Anand's mind went to those less fortunate. He continued the tradition of their childhood and always incorporated into their Christmas a project to distribute food to local communities.

Around the time the siblings became adolescents, it became apparent that things were tense between Anand's parents. The way Anand remembers it, his father wanted to accumulate and display their wealth, but his mother viewed it as a source of tension and was keen to have less and give away more. His siblings sided with their father and had no trouble finding ways to spend the family wealth over the years. Anand, like his mother, came to see the family wealth as more of a burden than a benefit.

> When there is absurd wealth, there is always a burden. The burden is not just on you because one must always remember others are lacking. Just look at India. You will see tremendous wealth and the poorest poor. Among the minted, there is a burden that manifests in despicable ways. You want for things that are completely unnecessary. You think you are shouldering the burden for society, but you forget the burden you create. You become so out of touch, what seems a kind gesture, a generous tip becomes an encounter that includes unnecessary critiques, your remarks are out of touch, and what you are willing to overlook is shameful.

Anand never forgot his nanny who passed away from polio, nor did his mother. As a teen, Anand overheard a tense conversation in which his mother lamented that they should have brought in medical support sooner, while his father said the money they gave to the nanny's family was sufficient to compensate for their loss. Anand's mother carried her sense of guilt regarding the nanny's death and Anand's physical difficulties with her to her grave, while his father died without having ever mentioned the incident after that conversation with his mother. At an age younger than Anand is now, his father developed dementia, losing most of his memories many years prior to his passing. Anand believes that, because of the many insensitive things his father did and said, perhaps his father's memory loss was lucky, too.

MIDLIFE CRISIS

After he graduated from Berkeley, Anand remained in the Bay Area and worked for a start-up company for several years. The job, coupled with the culture of the region, brought him a new sense of independence: "The Bay Area is brilliant if you're not able-bodied. Everyone there has something going on with their body or their mind is a bit off or both. It's ace if you're different. You certainly are not going to be made to feel like people are staring because you're differently abled. Might'a been timing in my life; in any event, that was when I really came into my own with walking."

The highlight of his time in the Bay Area was walking around enjoying the beautiful landscape with a forearm crutch. Developments with assistive devices and early self-monitoring technology helped boost Anand's mobility. Over the years, he tried numerous different types of mobility aids that helped him enjoy hiking and exploring nature on his own. While the region contains difficult terrain in the sense that there are hills and mountains with uneven ground, he found the generally good weather and natural beauty were sharp contrasts to the dreary environs of his youth.

Yes, Anand sometimes ran into trouble, sometimes exercising so strenuously that he could not regain control over his muscles and would be forced to give his body a reprieve for weeks at a time. He also fell often. Sometimes his falls put him in dangerous situations and he required help from a stranger. The strangers were usually kind and helpful. Once, he was mugged after having a bad fall; he wasn't further injured but had his wallet and keys stolen. Now he laughs about it, but losing these two essential items made it quite difficult for him to get home, and it was raining.

When Anand thinks back to his fall and the mugging, he reminds himself that it is okay to have a positive attitude about life. Around this time in his life, he had been living independently for many years. He was coming into his own professionally and physically, and continuing his spiritual journey with Hinduism. Anand spent a good amount of time thinking about and questioning his life and the way society is oriented. As an underlying optimist, this phase of life threw him. He felt out of sorts. He considered taking his own life.

> This was a difficult time. I was not young, but there were many things I had not experienced yet. I wanted to experience being with a woman. I saw how it was to move differently. You see different ways to live life. I questioned all the ways. I had to go through that questioning, that "midlife crisis." We all get stuck in the middle sometimes, and it can be difficult to make it to the other side. Time passed slowly then. . . . It was necessary for me to rethink my path and remember that it was all going to be just fine.

In what he describes as his "middle age," Anand began to question his path. He observed his two siblings and their growing families. He wondered why he didn't have a family of his own, even whether he wanted to continue his life in a body that was limited. At about this time, both of his parents passed away. This opened a sort of vacuum in which he began to question what would come next and considered his own aging for the first time.

Prior to his parents' deaths, Anand had been in the habit of speaking with them by phone several times a week. When his father died, Anand felt relief. He felt as if he had already lost his father to dementia years before. Anand perceived his father as a dismissive and controlling man, whose memory declines exacerbated his problems with anger management.

Within a year of his father's death, Anand's mother passed away, too. Of course, Anand could not have known she would pass away so soon after her husband of over sixty years. Anand thought he would step in to care for this kind woman when his father no longer could. He was instead distressed to realize that he could not make it work. His mother was not going to move from England to be cared for, and at this time Anand did not believe that he could manage himself physically outside the Bay Area. In retrospect, he realizes he probably had more options than he thought, but as Anand likes to say, "Hindsight is 20/20."

If he could go back to that time, the one thing Anand would tell himself to do differently would be to exercise. Certain parts of his body were always going to hurt. He was always going to have an excuse to give up and for a brief time, he did. In the years following the loss of his parents, Anand would find himself further distanced from his siblings in terms of their political views, family lifestyle choices, and many other ways except one—they all developed diabetes, which is interesting because of the lack of genetic connection between the siblings.

Unlike his siblings, Anand would reconnect to exercise within a few years of his parents' passings. His siblings grew less mobile over time, and Anand went in the opposite direction. At Christmas, even after their parents died, he would see his siblings and notice that, year by year, they came to lose their breath easily and have a harder time moving around. When Anand found himself at a stage in life where he could have given in to physical ailments permanently, he instead resolved to keep going and keep moving.

Anand's mother's physical decline raised intense feelings of resentment over his own physical limitations. Yes, he had experienced frustration and the occasional bout of envy, but nothing like this. He tortured himself with the fantasy that she ought to be able to depend on him to catch her if she tripped or just needed to steady herself by taking his arm. Instead, he was in his own unsteady body, a continent away in her later years. In retrospect, Anand put undue pressures on himself by holding unrealistic expectations. His mother never expected him to hold her up or catch her if she fell. She had the means to pay for caregivers. She even had the means to support Anand if he had chosen not to work. She lived her life in a way that was compassionate.

In those years of doubt, Anand would be at work surrounded by people and yet feel lonely and isolated. He began to dread activities that once felt fulfilling. His work and religious community provided a source of interaction, yet he struggled to connect. Anand claims that he was born an optimist and, up to this point, he had been patient, persistent, and focused on figuring out how to move forward. Part of what Anand now recognizes as a source of anguish was the realization that he was unlikely to marry or have children of his own. It was a time of transition in which he struggled with who he was. He says that he made the mistake of allowing pessimism to enter his life in a way that he has not tolerated since. This was the only time when Anand stopped exercising his body. Today, he generally thinks of this time as a period of upheaval in which he reconstructed his sense of self.

"ONE MUST ALWAYS PRACTICE BEING AN OPTIMIST"

Literature on the topic of optimism suggests that positive outcomes such as improved health and well-being are generally associated with having a positive and upbeat view on life. Anand is now resolved to channel that compassion toward himself, to be patient with himself and recognize that he has done a great job inhabiting and caring for his body. It took this "midlife crisis" for him to reconnect with his optimistic roots.[2]

In the year following his mother's death, Anand felt the desire to overcome his grief and combat his pessimism by volunteering in an elder-care home. Anand considers himself a person who lives his life in ways that differ from the majority and believes that his volunteer experience might be one way to demonstrate that. Anand loved being in the elder-care home. Although he is critical of elder homes as institutions, he knows that he will end up in one.

> I have visited many elder-care, convalescent, old-age homes—call them what you will. These places are full of people who are just moving differently than the rest of society. I see some of the people in there and they are much younger than me, just sitting there doing nothing. It is sad; it is a sad commentary on societies around the world that we like to just lock people away. Tuck them away so no one has to bother. It is sad; it really is. I'm not afraid for what comes in the next life but in this life, I know this is where I'm going to end up. Hopefully [I will] have someone nice who comes to talk with me.

He found the experience of volunteering in an elder-care home to be cathartic. He thoroughly enjoyed the company of several residents. Over time, through his friendships in the home, he came to think differently about his mother's final years. He came to realize that he was a kind and good son. He found peace in knowing that his mother was well cared for toward the end of her life. In time, he came to feel greater contentment in relation to her situation. He also came to realize that, while he does not fear his own death, he is in no hurry for it—there are many new challenges that he still looks forward to.

In the time that Anand refers to as his "midlife crisis," he also took an interest in animals. Anand got a beautiful service dog named Asha. Once he connected with Asha, Anand had no more experiences with being robbed. He also found that he was much less likely to trip or fall in Asha's presence. Asha was a tremendous source of comfort, as was reconnecting with his underlying optimism and the principles of Hinduism. Anand still finds comfort in the afterlife and in knowing that both he and his parents will each return to this earth as another living being in another life.

He also found comfort in a group that helps people experiencing grief connect with therapy horses. Later, he joined a group that brings together people with disabilities who are interested in being around and riding horses. In addition to helping change his outlook on life, being with horses renewed his focus on enhancing his physical mobility. It also led him to make the move to Germany.

Anand and I reconnected during the COVID-19 pandemic, when many old friends found one another again. He was living in Berlin and had just been released from the hospital. Again, he saw himself as one of the lucky ones. He viewed the pandemic as a wakeup call for the world, imagining that perhaps people would become aware of the world's inequities and political injustices. Although he sees that there is much to be concerned about, the pandemic was another opportunity for Anand to reaffirm his commitment to optimism.

Anand likes to say that "actions speak louder than words" and that "acts of kindness are more meaningful than kind words." This is why he has chosen to spend much of his life devoted to caring for other living beings. Animals intuitively understand when a person is trying to convey kindness and innately exude compassion.

Anand notes that people sometimes act differently toward him in direct relation to the fact that he walks and moves differently. He feels the stigma of moving differently and has experienced people who avoid interactions or eye contact simply for how he looks. Sometimes people speak to him as if he doesn't speak the language or is hard of hearing, which is ironic given his incredible facility with languages. Anand happens to be fluent in five languages and conversant in another two; sometimes, it's given him a chance to have some fun with those who treat him as if he has learning difficulties.[3]

Despite enjoying the climate and natural beauty of California, Anand decided to move to Germany for several reasons. He recognized that he needed a change in his life. He had a deep-rooted feeling that he was heading down a negative path, and it wasn't the life trajectory he wanted. He had grown bored of being around coworkers who were obsessed with wealth—they reminded him of his siblings. They were on a hedonic treadmill, constantly attaining more and constantly wanting more. Anand also fell into a political disagreement with a couple members of his religious community, which left him feeling that it was time to find a new community. He was interested in moving to the European Union, and Germany appealed to him because he already spoke the language and because it seemed that the country was trying to make amends for its past horrific treatment of people with disabilities. When an employment opportunity in Germany came to his attention, Anand started looking at communities that connected people with disability and horses and found one that seemed to be a good fit. He sensed he might find a new start there, even if he had to leave his support animal Asha behind.

The change of scenery turned out to be important. It helped Anand reset some of his neuropathways. In a new country with lots of new physical challenges, Anand didn't have time to dwell on negative thoughts. His mind was occupied by moving his body in his new space and making sure he didn't make too many mistakes or offend anyone with his rusty German at work.

> At that point, I had to decide whether to be guided by fear or by love. I know there is always a choice to let things go . . . between optimism and pessimism. I wake up with pain every day. I can choose to give into that. But no, I choose to do my exercises as I always have. I do this so that I can keep moving because if I gave in to the pain, well, then, that would be the end of me. I don't have the years ahead of me to restart or to risk another fall. I have to keep moving the way I move. The exercises keep me moving and they keep my head in the right space. I practice that, too. One must always practice being an optimist; it is a mistake to think that it just comes naturally.

As Anand adjusted to his newly adopted country, he renewed his vow to practice optimism and devoted more time to his exercise routines. In his sixties, Anand spends many of his weekends at the stables where he met Myrna, who has become his companion for well over a decade (they bonded initially when they witnessed a horse giving birth). Anand describes Myrna as sensitive, extremely kind, well read, and great with languages. He loves the way she understands him and shares his love for animals. Anand now has a companion dog named Luna who has a spring in its step that is similar to Asha's and who gets along very well with Myrna's service dog. Myrna and Anand have a great deal in common beyond the fact that they are both optimists and move differently than many other people. They also love Italian food, beer, and reading Russian novels in German.

MORE THAN A BODY

When Anand and I met at an outdoor café in Berlin, it had been more than twenty years since we had seen each other in person. It was lovely to see Anand and to meet Myrna and their dogs. The weather was fantastic, and the conversation flowed naturally. Lots of time had passed, we covered lots of ground, and we eventually settled on the topic of aging. There was a point in our conversation when Myrna explained that she had heard women complain that they feel invisible when they reach a certain age. Myrna never quite felt the sympathy for these women that they seemed to expect. We had been discussing aging and how perceptions change over time. Myrna laughed that she has a tiny violin to play for these women who once felt that they looked so good and now suffer for lack of attention. While she understands that society favors youthful beauty, she resents the self-pity that some women assert as they try to let you know how beautiful they once were.

Myrna eloquently described how she has always felt that beauty is better expressed with age. She herself feels more attractive as she approaches seventy than at any other point in her life. She finally appreciates her body for the things it can do and doesn't waste time worrying about the things it can't. She referred to feeling like she is finally "more than a body" and explained that, for most of her life, she could feel people's eyes on her because she stood out. Her wheelchair got in the way or needed to be moved out of the way or was somehow always in the way. Her body never looked like other bodies and didn't look the way people expected it to look.

Anand agrees with Myrna. He, too, is enjoying his body more at this stage, even in moments when he is acutely aware of the ways it is declining. Much of the early decades of his life were spent observing others engage fully in activities that were not open to him. Today, much more of the world has opened to him. He embraces being in his seventh decade, and he refuses to live in the liminal space between being alive and moving on to the next life. In the past, his body often drew unwanted attention when other people looked at him or had to interact with him. They didn't often understand how to engage with him, how to talk to him, or even how to embrace him. Now, he is making up for many lost embraces.[4]

Having grown up in a family that valued wealth, Anand particularly enjoys interacting with people in ways that are not focused on money or status. Instead, he enjoys connecting with people who are interested in finding the meaning and joy in life. He spends much of his time with Myrna—outdoors whenever possible. Things can be difficult logistically because Myrna needs help with some ADLs, including bathing, and during the pandemic it was sometimes difficult to find caregivers. For a period of several months, the couple lived together in Myrna's apartment, rarely going outside. It was then they learned that living together was not ideal for them. No, their ideal is to live in separate spaces and to enjoy each other's company every moment they are together.

Before he met Myrna, Anand had spent most of his life alone. But now, when he is unable to be with her, he experiences a new form of connection to the concept of loneliness. His world is connected to hers, whether they are together or apart. Although they prefer to have a living alone together (LAT) relationship, the time when Myrna was in the hospital was extremely difficult. In addition to feeling deep concern for her, Anand experienced a shift that made him realize his time left in the world would feel incomplete without her. They are now keen to make up for lost time, especially for that time that was spent at the hospitals and strictly indoors. They choose to sit outside as much as possible; spend time at the stables in the company of the horses; and do charitable work, both by serving on boards and by working with and supporting a group that creates opportunities with therapeutic horses. Of course, their time fills up with doctors' appointments and, most important, doing their regular exercises.[5]

The pandemic offered an interesting inversion in which Myrna and Anand observed their world expand; people previously outside the disability community experienced what it was like to be restricted or confined inside for prolonged periods of time, and some joined chat groups and virtual get-togethers for the first time. For Anand, the widening of the communities they had belonged to seemed like a blessing in the early days. He felt the promise that more people would understand what it was like to feel stymied by public infrastructure and health constraints. He remains optimistic that if more people connect within the disability community and understand the need for reinterpretations of access, options for socialization and public action will increase among people whose bodies don't operate like those in the mainstream.[6]

Anand believes that the greatest enhancement to their lives that came with the pandemic was the expansion of online exercise classes. Anand has always been technologically savvy and one step ahead when it came to communications and assistive devices, so when he praises something related to tech, you know he means it. The plethora of options they now have for exercising has meant a renewed sense of devotion to moving their bodies.

EXERCISE AS A RELIGION

In many ways, Anand's body compares favorably to other people around his age. Although he will never be able to roll out of bed and walk to the bathroom without some form of support, his body has become stronger over time in many ways. Like many other people, his body creaks and aches and requires maintenance. But because he has maintained the habit of exercising regularly, his body has held up better than others. The habits Anand has cultivated to make exercise a ritual to live by have helped him age successfully. So, too, has his sense of humor: "Wouldn't it be great if we got a new set of teeth in our fifties? Perhaps we could push a button that would temporarily eject our ears so we could give them a good cleaning out, and perhaps it would be beneficial to have an exit system for food around our stomach before the small intestine so we could discretely and painlessly get rid of food that doesn't sit well."

Anand lives by the principles of Hinduism, but he views exercise as his religion. For decades, failing only for a brief period in his midlife crisis, he has done his exercises first thing in the morning and again several times throughout the day. He subscribes to self-determination theory, which suggests that we are each motivated by the fulfillment of our needs and the desire to realize our full potential. He knows his body needs exercise to stay moving and that he is more likely to achieve his full potential by staying physically mobile. This does not mean that if he were more physically limited, as in Myrna's case, he would feel incapable of contributing. Instead, he believes that he is obligated to himself to make the most of the body he currently inhabits.[7]

Anand never wakes up and says, "I hope I feel motivated today." Instead, he gets up and he does his exercises. He subscribes to several online exercise programs and does all of Myrna's exercises with her, too. This is not because he is competitive or thinks she can't do it on her own but because he enjoys being with her and participating in her life in ways that support her strength.

In his current stage of life, when many people might resign themselves to moving less, Anand is optimistic that he and Myrna will retain their functional mobility. He knows exercise is the key to enhancing their life together. Being with Myrna reinforces his awareness of the need not to take functional mobility for granted. For this, he has many gadgets and devices to enhance and assist with their exercise habits.

> I love my devices. My phone can do things that I never dreamed possible. Our brains have changed to the point that we no longer need to remember anything, but if we use them correctly there are many ways our body can benefit. Remember when we had to memorize phone numbers? No more, Michelle! I tell you, now our brains are mush. We really don't need to retain information any longer. But the body must continue functioning even if the mind is mush. My devices help me do everything; they help me walk; they monitor my body. I spend a good deal of time working with software to help increase my range of motion and address my strength imbalance. I can actively work on certain muscles in very

precise ways before I develop an injury. My devices can even try to make me wake up and feel like moving.

As a student of economics, the so-called dismal science, Anand knows that there are always trade-offs in life. When he purchases a new piece of exercise equipment, he knows that the money could have gone to a charity. When he decides to use his energy to meet someone in a café, he knows that he could have saved that energy to do his exercises. The only thing that he sees as having no consequences to himself or any negative externalities is doing his exercises. Doing his exercises and getting Myrna do hers as well is likely to keep them both out of the hospital longer. They are careful and have learned how to avoid injury when they move.

Yes, the dismal science—remember, I am an optimist. The dismal science teaches that there is always an opportunity cost of your time. You can go to graduate school to study economics or you can take that time and work and earn money, right? But the opportunity cost of not exercising—that is important. We have people who can't be bothered to go make their bodies move because they don't want to take time away from work. What happens when the body stops exercising? It stops working. Now don't get me started on people who are starving and whatnot. The inequality around the world is despicable. . . . There are different approaches from an economic development standpoint that we can examine there, but coming back to exercise, this is important. Yes, it is a first-world concern, but I tell you, when you are dealing with hospital systems that must be shared and people of varying status rely on, well, then, it is very important that we each take care to maintain our bodies the best we can. A body that is exercised regularly is going to do better in terms of recovery from surgery and in terms of recovery from a fall. And a person who is self-actualized will do what they can to take care of their body. When more people do this, this means more time professionals can tend to those in need; potentially it means more resources to allocate to other problems.

Anand is taken by Maslow's theory of self-actualization and views exercise as an important component of reaching actualization. He has achieved most of his fundamental needs, including self-esteem, belonging, safety, nourishment, and shelter. Each is connected to his ability to exercise. Anand is concerned that there are few external incentives for people to exercise, particularly later in life. Many people find it hard, he pointed out, especially if they haven't done it regularly, and so there needs to be supports and encouragement and possibly even economic incentives to get people to exercise—maybe vouchers, discounts, gifts, or subsidies. People note opportunity costs of exercising when it comes to the opportunity cost of their time. It is certainly true that cowboys, ranchers, manual laborers, and people who move at work all day do not need to make extra time to exercise. Many of us, however, cannot afford *not* to find ways of exercising our bodies.[8]

For a boy who was told he would never walk, Anand has made a lot of strides. Anand knows that aging is hard. He sometimes finds that he must remind himself that he is an optimist. For most of his life, he has exuded a sense of calm and kindness that makes you want to be around him. He believes that the best way to combat aging is to remove the idea that any particular phase will last forever.

Indeed, the optimist sees a bad situation and says, "This won't last forever." Well, that is how I look at aging: it won't last forever. Yes, even you will die and I will die. I live a better life because I don't fear what comes next. I see what is happening and I look at the alternatives. The mother I was born to, she would have struggled to put food on the table. The family I grew up in put food on many family tables. To make this day good, you must have worked and exercised yesterday.

Anand uses what he has and does what he can, as the quote from Arthur Ashe at the start of this chapter suggests. His lifestyle incorporates regular exercise in ways that have allowed him to keep physically mobile—more so today sometimes than his able-bodied peers. He has the confidence to understand that he needs to exercise his body in ways that are sustainable and not be bothered by other people's judgments about the way his body looks or moves.

The lessons Anand imparts include learning to be compassionate with yourself and cultivate optimism. Keeping trying: try new things; try different ways of thinking about what it means to have a functional body; and try different ways of being caring toward others because when others need you, it can be good motivation to take care of yourself. Find groups that support your interests; find devices and supports that work for your body. Don't spend your life fearing death, don't underestimate the importance of having a change of scenery, and don't underestimate the power of an exercise routine.

As a mature man, Anand observes how some of his peers, who are new to movement challenges, struggle. He sees himself as lucky to have had so many years of training with his body. There are days when Anand is so happy that he actually fears dying because he worries his next life won't be as good as this one, which was so full of privileges. To be around Anand is a lesson in the importance of optimism.

7

COMMITMENT

You always have two choices: your commitment versus your fear.
—Sammy Davis Jr.

With his toned body and upright posture, Felipe is a handsome and athletic man. I often found myself straightening up in Felipe's company—even when we were talking virtually—because I could tell he was sitting up straight, aligned and alert. In conversation, he interrupts readily, although never rudely, and enjoys inserting his experiences or the experience of someone he knows into any conversation. Felipe is always looking to make connections, to make you feel that you share something in common, and try to make you better. He is kind and energetic, with the sort of keenness that makes me realize some people never relax.

Felipe doesn't let anything slow him down, and it would be hard to know he lives with chronic pain. He hides the fact that parts of his leg and lower back constantly radiate a dull pain. When he walks or moves even slightly, the pain sometimes shoots into other regions of his body, causing excruciating bouts of intense pain. Felipe is a proponent of pushing through pain, however; instead of retreating to bed, Felipe is a high-functioning master athlete who exercises regularly. He's also a lot of fun to be around.

Both serious and playful, Felipe was the youngest of his siblings. At this point, he has outlived all five of his brothers and his sister. Born into the favelas of Brazil, where he was discovered at age five, he spent most of his childhood and adolescence living away from home, training in judo. Felipe's childhood was primarily focused on being a competitive athlete. He holds multiple identities, and with age, he has come to see that each compliments the other.

> I like to refer to myself as Afro-Brazilian Pardo: Preto with a twist of Indio. Actually, best way I like to put it is I'm like a Neapolitan ice cream! I'm from all over, been all over, because I traveled starting very young with judo. Everybody thinks I'm from somewhere else, and, of course, I can speak many languages. The funny thing to me is when someone is convinced I'm from where they are from—they can't recognize that I am actually born very far away.

I first met Felipe in Toronto when he was in town for an international athletic event. I didn't know it at the time, but he was also in town to pay an old boyfriend a visit. During his month-long trip, a colleague introduced us and suggested Felipe should talk to me about his experience as a retired athlete. Felipe immediately retorted that he did not identify as a "retired" anything, but he was up for talking about his experience as an elite athlete and coach. He also had some advice to share with me: straighten up!

The first thing he said when we met for our interview was that he worried I wasn't maximizing my potential in terms of how I carry my body. To Felipe, it is essential to carry the body with poise and strength. He would remind me many times that "the muscles must support the bones and the bones must be strong." It was the first of many tips he'd give me about the skin, the body, and aging in general.

THE SELFISH ATHLETE

The bulk of Felipe's childhood was spent training and traveling between training locations and his family home. Felipe started his judo training after he was spotted by a coach while playing in the streets, and he showed tremendous potential. He was fit and agile, with body control and strength beyond his years. He also had the right temperament for a potential judoka. Felipe was a daredevil, not afraid of inserting himself into a fight or jumping off steep ledges. He also demonstrated poise and a keen intellect at a young age. He had a sense of curiosity, sometimes wandering off on his own, but Felipe was also easy to reel back in and was eager to follow instruction. He was self-focused, motivated by praise, and willing to give his all.

One bad memory illustrates his tendency to wander and the path he might have ended up on. It also provides some context for the tensions within his family. When he was six years old, Felipe fell behind two of his brothers and ended up wandering on his own as they made their way home after a pickup game in the neighborhood. By the time his brothers found Felipe, he had gotten into a bit of trouble. If only his brothers had shown up just a few minutes later, Felipe is convinced they would have found him getting along well with the child. The moment his brothers arrived, however, Felipe was in the midst of a fight, being grabbed and held in the air by a man. He'd taken a toy from the man's child, and the man intervened. But the man was barely older than Felipe's eldest brother, and somehow a fight ensued. Felipe's middle brother was brutally boxed in the ear, leaving him deaf on one side, and he came away with a lifelong scar snaking from his ear to his chin.

To hear Felipe tell the story is to hear a colorful depiction of the favelas of Brazil mixed with a restrained account of a world full of danger and limited opportunities. In the time Felipe was growing up and until 1970, the average woman in Brazil gave birth to at least five children (now the fertility rate in Brazil is under two). His home lacked electricity and running water; the family lived in what could best be described as one room with a roof and less than ideal walls.

At around eight years old, Felipe moved to be near a judo training facility. He lived in an apartment with a coach and other boys near his age. To this day, he remembers how proud he felt for being selected for this special opportunity. His mother cried, but his father insisted this was important. Felipe sensed that it was his obligation to go and to do well. He was destined to be a judoka. He always had a feeling in the pit of his stomach, however, that he was different. He missed being with his brothers, he was intellectually curious and had minimal exposure to schooling, and he was aware at a young age that he was not sexually interested in girls. He preferred boys.[1]

So Felipe always felt "off," but he was never homesick or bored. Felipe always had the sense he could be replaced at any moment, and he felt on edge to perform his best. Even though he was very young when he first left home to train, he could tell judo was his ticket to a different life. Part of his journey was distancing himself from his family. He was aware sometimes that his brothers resented him for being the one chosen. One brother even told Felipe that it was actually their older brothers who caught the scout's eye—Felipe was chosen only because he was the youngest.

Perhaps the biggest point of distancing came when Felipe was around ten years old and his family experienced a trauma that changed each of them forever. While Felipe was living away near the training facility, a group of men broke into the space where his family lived. They injured his father and brothers, and they killed his sister. Felipe returned home for the funeral, but from that point on, he only visited about once a year. His only sister had suffered untold pain, and his family would never recover. But Felipe had not been there, and he was so young. There was so much he didn't understand. He decided that it would be best to focus on being the best, in the hopes his success in judo would bring joy to his family. In retrospect, he learned that many of his brothers interpreted his drive as a selfish abandonment of the family.

Looking back, Felipe acknowledges that he was very young when his sister was killed and not truly capable of consoling his family over what had happened while he was away. His family embraced their Christianity, but it was of little comfort to Felipe. Judo was his religion. Training required his full attention—it was demanding and rewarding and, most of all, it gave him something to focus on.

THE COMMITTED ATHLETE

Felipe had what can be considered a relatively long athletic career. He was an incredibly committed athlete who endured many injuries, but he was disciplined and performed well. Over the years, Felipe represented his country at several Olympic Games as well as world championships and other prestigious tournaments. Felipe is that rare person who went to the Olympics and had a good time. Perhaps this was because he was able to go more than once, but it is more likely because his personality was inclined to allow him to enjoy and get the most out of his experience.

In most sports, winning requires full concentration—this is certainly true in judo. Life outside judo cannot be too distracting. Before each competition, Felipe had a ritual he would go over in his head, a cleansing process whereby he erased certain critical thoughts. This ritual was essentially a review of his neural pathways so that they would wire properly. He describes it as a sort of forced out-of-body experience that allowed him to step back, assess where he was, remove distraction, and focus on the task ahead. Felipe would then take control of his body to ensure it moved the way he needed it to.

> Here's the thing, I know what it's like to win, to feel I did it right. It is important to see how all that work paid off. Of course, I also know what it's like to lose; it is something very important. I think it's a myth that people believe you'll always remember your glory days—I think the thing people actually most remember [are] the mistakes they made in their glory days. The goal in your glory days is to focus entirely on one thing; you put all your eggs in one basket and then the basket is ripped from under you. That is powerful because the win feels really good. But you must remember that you will fall out of the spotlight, you will always be replaced, and what you have left is whatever you choose to remember.

Anything that might take away from an ideal competition must be eliminated or put on hold. For many years, Felipe filled his mind only with thoughts of competition, channeling all his experiences into the next win. He would go over his past victories, cataloguing the moves needed to accomplish more, and he would ruminate on losses, looking for what went wrong so that he wouldn't repeat the mistake. He would also relive negative experiences from his life and, as though watching a film on loop, search them for ways to channel himself toward competition.

Felipe was in his thirties when he retired from competition. Unlike many athletes whose careers end with major injury, Felipe ended his career on his own terms—for the most part.

> Yes, it was hard to stop, hard to realize, "Okay, yeah, this is over. That is the end of that very big, very important part of my life." I was committed, I *am* committed to judo. To me it is a part of who I am. I gave everything to the sport. Yes, I had a long career. If I was in a different sport, if I had ever taken it straight to my head, wiped out completely, if I was a woman—there is no way I could have competed that long. If I was a woman, they would have sent me packing at a point that for me I was only just having things coming together. I used all those experiences as a coach, but I was in too long. Not many people will say this.

Felipe believes he was encouraged to continue competing longer than what might have been appropriate. Fellow athletes were cut because of major injury, encouraged to stop in order to further their education, or offered support to find a placement in military service or launch their careers. (Women were not offered these opportunities.) Felipe was encouraged to continue competing because he was very good, he managed to avoid major injury, and he maintained a firm commitment to staying in the game. He also stayed on because his coaches wanted to keep him on and Felipe didn't have a concept of what else to do: "I would never permit someone to stay as long as I did. It was still hard for me, don't get me wrong, but there had been many times the doctors looked at me and said, 'Okay, you have this injury, what do you want to do?' They would check with me and my coach. And, of course, I would say, 'Let's keep going,' and so we did."

So Felipe's retirement was *relatively* easy. Being replaced is rarely a pain-free experience. It was time to call it quits after a less-than-ideal world championship game. While he was competing, Felipe had no idea it would be his last competition. Today, however, it is clear to him that he was no longer in top form. His timing was off and his head was not in the right place. The regular mental cleansing ritual Felipe had relied on for years was no longer working. And Felipe had finally found a relationship with a man who captured his heart. In truth, he was ready to move on to other chapters in life.

Felipe had a talk with his coach on their way home from the world championships, and it seemed his coach had already moved on. Within a day of Felipe's last competition, his coach announced Felipe's replacement. He offered to connect Felipe with another coach who might take him on as an assistant coach but had very little to offer in terms of how to cope with the physical and mental transition from being an elite athlete.[2]

"EVERYONE IS REPLACEABLE"

The first few months were rough. Felipe's body and mind reacted in drastic ways. He knew that he wanted to retire. He was past his prime, but he still had a desire to feel important and to be included. He likens it to the feeling of wanting to be invited to a party you don't actually want to attend.

He became an outsider when it came to elite sports. He missed connecting closely with others based on their shared interests. He also missed having an audience. After having been primed to focus on himself, Felipe felt lonely in the early days of his retirement. He would find himself on the verge of tears when getting a haircut or in the shower, doing ordinary things. When it all came to a halt, he felt empty.

After nearly twenty years of never taking more than a day off from training, Felipe had grown accustomed to his rigid exercise and eating regimens. It took only a few days away from training to feel all the pent-up energy bubbling within. At first, it made him feel alive. But his feelings vacillated between relief at not having any commitments, anger toward his coach, and sorrow for having lost what he had achieved as a competitor. Throughout, he mourned lost relationships.

Being an elite judoka was an identity Felipe had come to embody in every aspect. When that part of his life ended, he questioned who he was. He had observed other athletes who retired, but when they did, they tended to disappear entirely and were immediately replaced. Felipe always figured that he would be unique because he had always felt unique. He thought his own retirement would be different, although, in reality, he had very little sense of what it would be like and what was to follow in his life.

In the first year of his athletic retirement, Felipe spent a fair amount of time drinking, dating, and living a life that he never permitted himself earlier. Still consuming the calories of an athlete but living like a party boy, he put on weight and felt sluggish, tired, and restless. Felipe relocated several times, taking up residence in various European cities. He also tried moving back to Brazil, but it wasn't a good fit. It was a moment when many of Felipe's friends and family were established in their work and families; all but one of his brothers had married, one had already remarried. They had children, and Felipe enjoyed his nieces and nephews, but he felt estranged from his parents and brothers. Too much time had passed, too many experiences had been missed. Felipe was an outsider to his own family.

Felipe would eventually create his own family, but the distance he felt between the family he was born into would always cause him pain. He wants to remember himself as a good brother, but he feels that his identity as a child was above all as an athlete: "I think the main experience of being a high-performance athlete, it teaches you many wonderful things: discipline, humility, how to be strong. Also you must be selfish. And you must remember: everyone is replaceable."

When Felipe moved away from his family as a child, his space in the home was immediately taken over by another brother. In fact, as soon as he moved out, it was as if he had never lived in his home. He was replaced quickly on the national team, too, but the same could not be said within the world of judo. His name remains in the records; his legacy not only as a competitor but also as a coach is indelible.

"I ONCE WAS BEAUTIFUL"

After Felipe retired from athletic competition, he landed an assistant coaching job, which kept him busy and involved regular travel. As he focused on training young judoka, his own exercising ceased. He realizes now that his life was lacking because he did not have his own goals. He spent many days at work just phoning it in, not feeling a strong sense of individual purpose. He missed having his own chase for victory and being on the team. He loved being a coach and providing guidance, but it can be hard watching from the sidelines when you know the rush of being in the spotlight.

He also felt the aftermath of years of being thrown to the floor and having fingers broken from grip fighting. These activities take a toll on the body. The intensity required to perform at the elite level meant that Felipe had strained his knees and lower back, and likely added stress to his joints in ways that have made it painful to walk since his thirties. In his early retirement, several years passed without Felipe giving much regard to his physical fitness. As an assistant coach, he worked, ate, and slept as he pleased. Now outside the spotlight, he had the freedom, time, and money to enjoy dates with different men—he no longer had to hide his homosexuality completely.

In his thirties, Felipe used the pain he experienced in his joints to remind himself to find bodily pleasure. He enjoyed the gay dance scene where he could find it. In the late 1970s, he landed jobs in Paris and San Francisco and found himself moving to cities that offered more for gay men. In most of the world, homosexuality remained illegal, and being gay was something to hide. The gay community was excluded from mainstream life, and there were no gay-friendly places to live, but it was not difficult to find someone to be with if you were beautiful and in the right club.

Felipe enjoys reminiscing about his party days, when he lived to find a new club, especially a gay dance club. Under the watchful eye of coaches and family, he had been closeted for much of his life. Now he felt the need to make up for lost time. When Felipe was dancing, he felt like all his aches and pains went away. His true nature is to be competitive and when he was on the dance floor in the discos, Felipe wanted to be the most admired man in the room.

To be in the company of beautiful men who admired him and wanted to be with him was like a dream come true; that is, until the dream turned into a nightmare, and this carefree phase of life came to an end. As Felipe eloquently explained, "I once was beautiful. At one time, I danced until the music stopped. I knew what it was like to feel admired. I like that, you know. I like feeling beautiful. I was dazzling, and I was willing to risking everything to be near the dazzle of the sun."

It was hard to tell, as Felipe spoke these words, whether he was being wistful about his time as a competitive athlete or his days as a single man before he met his life partner, Alex. In some sense, I think it is the latter. Being gay then was risky, as it can be now. Many people reacted ignorantly and violently to the very idea of men who loved men. Felipe's party days also overlapped with the early years of human immunodeficiency virus (HIV) and acquired immunodeficiency syndrome (AIDS), and his close friend and sexual partner, Will, died. The couple was never monogamous (today, their relationship would likely be considered polyamorous), and they were open with each other about having sex with other men. But Felipe reminisces, "When it's about the body you're attracted to, you miss all sorts of red flags." Felipe now questions his need earlier in life for attention from other men, at times suggesting that it led him to unhealthy behaviors.

THE LONELY DEATH

Felipe learned that Will had AIDS, explained to him at the time as "gay-related immune deficiency (GRID)," only after Will died. Will's death was a very painful experience for Felipe. It brought back painful memories of his sister's death, and it took years before Felipe could be sure he didn't also have HIV or AIDS.

During this time, he confronted the realization that his life would not go on forever. Up to that point in his life, Felipe had felt ambitious and restless. He might not have always had a clear picture of his future; however, he *had* assumed his life would go on forever. Now he felt resentful, angry, and scared that he had been reckless and naïve. Until he learned about AIDS, he also considered being homosexual his own private concern. With the

AIDS crisis, he witnessed the world suddenly take a horrific interest in his community. Felipe observed the world as homophobic and moralistic. The gay community was blamed for the virus and, by some, for all the evils of the world.[3]

In addition to Rock Hudson, Cazuza, and Renato Russo, who sadly lost their lives to the virus, Felipe lost many friends around the world to AIDS.[4] During the AIDS crisis, many people died lonely deaths. The gay community, which took him in and adored him when judo all but discarded him, was being ripped apart. There was no reprieve from the sense of dread and threat. The way Felipe describes it, it took time for his group of friends to understand that condoms could reduce the risk of HIV infection, to learn how to manage their new reality. He experienced what he refers to as his "less-than-healthy phase," when each sexual experience could have meant acquiring HIV.

When Felipe was thirty-five, his father died of a heart attack. His mother begged him to come home for the funeral. In his family home and in his "less-than-healthy phase," Felipe looked in the mirror and suddenly he didn't recognize himself. His clothes didn't fit and his hair was receding. There were fine lines around his eyes and dark circles beneath them. His self-image had always featured having a good, strong body, but the man in the mirror didn't look (or feel) so good. Suddenly, his competitive instincts returned.

Felipe sometimes questions traditional ideas about masculinity. He did so at his father's funeral and does so when he thinks about his brothers. They were aggressive and inconsiderate. They were quick to fight and quick to anger; in their own way, they were sensitive and limited in their understanding of the world. None traveled outside Brazil, and none ever reached out to ask Felipe about his life. For all these reasons and more, Felipe always felt like an outsider among his brothers. Perhaps being gay added to Felipe's estrangement.

After his father's funeral, Felipe set out to change everything about his lifestyle. He started with his diet. His body reacted well to eliminating meat, so he ate only plant-based foods. Once he started to feel better about his appearance, he started swimming regularly. He had always loved the water, and swimming provided relief from his pain. His motivation for exercising shifted from needing to be in shape to compete to wanting to be in shape as a way of taking care of himself.

As an athlete and as a single man looking to enhance his dating life, Felipe had used his body without regard for its long-term sustainability. He made the decision to look after his body. It was a dramatic shift. With judo, Felipe was used to being in situations that he had to learn how to get out of. He used this skill to change his habits and create a lifestyle that better suited his interest in maintaining a longer life.

By the time that Earvin "Magic" Johnson, one of the most famous athletes in basketball, announced that he had HIV in 1991, Felipe had changed his lifestyle dramatically. In 1992, AIDS became the leading cause of death for American men between the ages of twenty-five and forty-five, and tennis star Arthur Ashe tested positive for HIV. At that point, Felipe was living in Quebec, "out of the closet," and in a loving relationship with Alex. He was working as an athletic coach, maintaining a vegetarian diet, and managing his pain primarily by swimming regularly.

Once Felipe got into swimming, his athletic tendencies kicked in. He proved to be a talented swimmer and, by his late forties, he was swimming in a competitive amateur league, which eventually led to decades as a master athlete. Felipe maintains that he has always been an athlete. That part of his identity never left him, although it might have fallen into the shadows at times.

Now as he enters his eighth decade and returns to the water, he still considers himself an athlete to his core.

Felipe is not shy about the fact that he had many sexual partners during his time as a single man. His athletic prowess led him to be studied in his approach to dating. Not only did Felipe keep track of the numbers of men he had been with, he kept a list of the kind words men said to him over the years. I have never seen this secret record, but I imagine it is handwritten in Portuguese, perhaps in a book tattered at the edges after all the years.

Felipe sometimes thought subconsciously that the more men he slept with, the more he would be remembered when he died. He came to realize, however, that having sex was not the only way he wanted to be remembered. Felipe had spent years questioning whether AIDS would claim his life and what his legacy would be. He always thought that his athletic records would live on, but he worried that his relationship to the athletic community was somewhat weak, and he knew his relationship with his family was strained.

LIVING YOUNGER

Felipe calls Alex the biggest influence in his life. Felipe and Alex met in a grocery store in Paris. They were near the produce, and Felipe questioned whether a particular apple was good to eat. Alex recommended a different one and gently brushed his hand against the middle of Felipe's back. That was all it took.

Being with Alex made Felipe realize that he wanted to be in a monogamous relationship for the rest of his life. Alex was someone Felipe wanted to take care of and someone he wanted to continue to be healthy for. In some ways, it was so simple.

Alex was always going to ask Felipe how his day had been, and he really cared about that day. Alex cared about all the rest of Felipe's days.

> It was somewhat suddenly important to me to be in a relationship with someone who really knew me and really loved me. Before [Alex], I imagined my own death, alone. Yes, there is a rush of excitement that comes with new relationships. But those are short-lived. Now I understand, new fast relationships are for people who can't figure out to make long-term relationships work, or a quick fix. Finding peace with being a person who wants commitment—that is the healthiest thing I've done.

Now in his eighties, Felipe still gets butterflies from two thoughts: his days competing at the world championships and the day he met Alex. One aspect of his relationship that Felipe sometimes feels conflict about, however, is that Alex is over a decade younger. Some of the conflict may come from the fact that Felipe was the youngest of his brothers and has always viewed himself as the baby. Felipe finds himself thinking about his age often: sometimes in relation to his father and brothers, sometimes in relation to Alex, sometimes in relation to his younger self or the expectations he feels imposed by gay culture.

It would be unfair to say that gay male culture is obsessed with recapturing youth, but sometimes Felipe feels that the community places a value on youthful beauty that can be difficult to live up to. Until his mid-forties, Felipe's perceptions of aging had been somewhat underdeveloped, and suddenly he longed to find ways to hold on to his youthfulness.

> Being gay, there are so many pressures on how one looks. Being an old, gay person of color—you have to feel good about yourself

to look good. You have to be confident to ignore it when people are like, "Oh, he's doing that." You know, being outside the norm in multiple ways can be a multiple whammy. There's stigma. So is being the older one in the relationship. Yes, I know people look at me, and I have to work harder to make sure I look like I still have "it." Before [Alex], I had another relationship with a younger man. I remember feeling glad he could see what remained of my youth and thinking, "This is good. He'll remember it when we grow old together." I held this fantasy that our time together was a touchpoint for the future. Of course, he had no concept of cataloguing my youth or my future plans for us to be together—he had no future plans for anything. And then when we broke up—I suddenly got old, very dramatically. I went hard-core into seeking out ways to be viewed as more attractive. I wore eyeliner then.

As a way to build strength and maintain body function as he aged, Felipe added weight lifting and stretching to his regular regime—practices he continues to this day. Felipe is wary of the additional marginalization that comes with being an old gay person of color. The best way he finds to combat marginalization is to stay fit. Although he is not a fan of identity politics and enjoys commenting on the ways the world has become more sensitive in ways that he finds unnecessary and unappealing, Felipe is mindful about his present stage in life. He knows that his time is limited simply because of his age, although he is quick to joke that, from now on, he will live only in countries with long life expectancies for men.

Felipe sometimes frets over being with a younger man, but he is also playful about being the older man in his relationship. Being with a younger partner helps Felipe feel motivated to stay in shape. Although Alex is significantly younger, he has been in poor health since they met, and his health has declined significantly since. It has been many years since Alex participated in the paid workforce because of his weakened respiratory system. But Felipe, who is the provider and caregiver in their relationship, loves taking care of Alex.[5]

Felipe believes that couples who exercise together will grow old together, and so he encourages Alex to exercise. He schedules time for them to lift weights or stretch together, and he regularly looks up fitness routines that are appropriate for Alex's condition and can be done in short bursts of time. Felipe says, "Sometimes I tell [Alex], 'You are my trophy boy. I am ancient in gay years.' I know he finds my thoughts ridiculous, but I see that other people see the age difference. For us, there is a divide when it comes to our age, even though I know I am aging better, but that is because I am very health-focused."

As an athlete, Felipe uses his chronic pain to keep moving. From his earlier years, he knows many people who pushed themselves to the limit physically and their bodies gave out. He has had friends who were extreme sports enthusiasts who died seeking thrills or the limits of human potential. Felipe is clear that he feels content that he achieved his potential early in life and at this point seeks contentment by working to sustain his strength.

Felipe wants to find ways to live younger. He loves to read about strength training techniques and to give advice. Each time we meet in person, he excitedly suggests what I need to do to present myself better. His advice consistently includes swimming, daily yoga, stretching, weight lifting, and regularly thinking about how to distribute the weight in my body evenly. Each is a practice dear to Felipe, honed over the course of at least five decades.

TIMING IS EVERYTHING

In sports like swimming, the winner is easy to determine: the winner is the one who makes it to the other end of the pool fastest and without receiving a disqualification. In judo, timing is also crucial, but the rules are a bit more complex. The present regulation time for men's judo is five minutes. Within that time, points are scored for each of three different types of throws. An *ippon* is awarded when an opponent is held down for twenty seconds (less if he gives up or passes out sooner). A *wasa-ari* is awarded for immobilizing an opponent for at least fifteen seconds but no more than twenty seconds. And a *yuko* is a type of throw where the winner is awarded in several ways, including by immobilizing an opponent for at least ten but no more than fifteen seconds.

Sometimes described as the "football of the martial arts," judo is highly technical and full contact, and takes years to learn. A successful judoka must be highly attentive to detail and willing to take risks. In other sports, it is typical to see progress within months, but it can take years to make significant progress in judo. The training is physically rigorous, and the scrutiny is intense. Every move matters when opponents engage. Although the difference between winning and losing can come down to only slight movements, the feeling of victory is enormous. Judoka can find it difficult to control themselves and express humility because each win stems from an extensive amount of training and comes with the possibility of lucrative endorsements from athletic companies, places on national teams, or jobs training others.

While the victories that come in judo are sweet, they are hard to come by. Most judoka lose more than they win. For this reason, Felipe sees loss as an essential piece of becoming masterful in any arena. He values each fall as an experience that made him stronger. He sees failure as an essential step toward winning. Each injury that he has endured broke him down, he says, but made him stronger in body and mind. As he approaches his later years, he values his own experiences with loss because they have helped him get stronger and feel more comfortable with his uncomfortable thoughts about death and legacy.

In the early days of the COVID-19 pandemic, Felipe sent me an email suggesting that a deep sense of loneliness had returned to him. He was concerned that the coronavirus would take Alex's life and about the many ways the virus and the lockdowns compromised his life. It reminded him of the early years of his athletic retirement. In both phases, Felipe felt a forced isolation and disconnect from the world as he knew it: "I feel like I did then, that the world is not what I thought it was. I wasn't prepared for this and am alternating between feeling an overwhelming sense of doom and then a familiar feeling of just being cut off from what I have grown accustomed to."

Alex's respiratory condition limited them only slightly in the years leading up to the pandemic, and Felipe and Alex had enjoyed an active social life. Felipe had been working in an administrative capacity for a national judo team and swimming with a master's swim club when the pandemic brought the world to a halt. Now the couple became extremely cautious. For many years, they stayed at home, and the only other people they saw were delivery workers who were received with double masks and lots of fear. Anyone else was seen only by online video and heard via old-fashioned phone calls.

Felipe retired completely and stopped all group exercise activities for two years. When I saw him in person in Tel Aviv, where he and Alex found themselves living at the start of the pandemic, he had returned to swimming. He said that *this* phase reminded him of around the time after his athletic retirement. It is hard to get back into to shape after taking time away from exercise. In his eighties, Felipe figures it is unlikely he will ever be able to swim as fast as he once did. But he's not worried about his speed—at this point, exercise is about managing pain and keeping his body moving—nor is he worried that his master's swim team will replace him. Nonetheless, fifty years later, the resentment over being so easily replaced as a judoka still stings.

AGING IS NOT FOR WIMPS

Felipe reminds me to sit up straight and to carry my body in a more balanced way. He also likes to remind me that even the best athletes experience more losses than wins. In his serious moments, he understands that there is virtue in the experience of loss and learning to live with the grief that accompanies major loss. When his sister was killed, Felipe learned to channel his pain into a commitment to judo, but he never fully processed the loss of his sister until his mother passed away.

Felipe's mother remains his role model when it comes to how he wants his own aging to be perceived. To her dying day, his mother was beautiful and kind. Although she carried a heavy burden in her heart, she was loving and resilient, precisely the kind of strong person Felipe hopes that he models through his actions. As an elite athlete and athletic coach, Felipe has strived to find sustainable ways to manage pain. For his legacy, he wants to exemplify strong and healthy aging. He looks to his mother as the epitome of aging with beauty and grace. When she passed away, Felipe was overcome with grief. Alex had only met her once—something Felipe regrets.

Although he has never fully embraced Christianity, Felipe reminds himself not to give into fear or temptation. He chooses love and commitment. The quote that starts this chapter suggests that there are always two choices in life. You can choose to be afraid, or you can choose to be committed. In his darkest hours, Felipe chose commitment. He left his family as a young boy to become an athlete. When his sister died, he chose to commit to his sport. When his sporting career ended, he chose to recommit to the world of sport as a coach. When he was afraid AIDS might claim his life, he chose to commit to a lifestyle he believed would lead to healthier days ahead. As he embraces his last chapters, he has chosen to commit himself to taking care of Alex and taking care of his body in healthy and sustainable ways: "As an athlete, I know how to be committed and how to adapt when need be. For [Alex] I have created a self-determined exercise routine. This took me years to develop. No—decades to develop. I'm gonna patent it. You can buy it. I developed it for [Alex] because this is what we need to keep ourselves strong."

Felipe finds strength in fighting rather than giving in to his own chronic pain and in caring for Alex. When I visited them in Tel Aviv, it was clear their relationship is strong, and they are determined to keep going for each other. In spite of this, there is a great deal of uncertainty in their lives. It is unclear where they will live next. Alex struggles at times to breathe without the aid of a portable machine. Felipe pointed out that he himself has already lived past the average life expectancy for a man in most regions of the world.

At our last visit, I couldn't help sensing that Felipe was trying to prepare me for the fact that he won't live forever. He is determined to keep going in order to be there for Alex for as long as possible. But Felipe has spent a good deal of time contemplating his own mortality recently.

Early in life, Felipe had the benefit of becoming really good at something, but it couldn't last forever. Over the years, Felipe has trained hundreds of high-performance athletes. He understands how to detect whether someone is teachable, whether they have the right temperament to make it as an elite athlete or whether they might be better served taking up sports as a hobby. Felipe's life has taken many turns, sometimes down less healthy pathways. In the instances where he faced the possibility of his own demise, he chose to assert control over his life by changing his path. He refuses to return to the closet or to live an ambiguous existence. Instead, Felipe embraces his homosexuality and attends to creating a long, healthy life for himself and his partner.

The lessons he imparts include learning to care for your body early and learning to carry yourself well. Posture is important to Felipe; he notes how important it is to have good posture when training and exercising, and he notes the importance of paying attention to your posture at all points in life. He illustrates the significance of learning to cope with loss and coming to terms with the fact that everyone is replaceable. Felipe also demonstrates how critical it is not to count on basking in your glory days. Instead, consider that you might learn the most from your past failures and feel more rewarded from living in the present. Felipe found it important to include different types of exercises in his repertoire; he swims, does yoga, lifts weights, and walks regularly. Don't assume you will live forever. Create your own sense of family, forgive yourself, and above all commit to yourself.

Felipe embraces the finitude of the human body while simultaneously fighting his pain and the inevitable deterioration that comes with age by exercising his body regularly. As we age, he notes, we become more aware of our physical limitations and also of the limitations of our memories. After decades of reflection, Felipe has concluded definitively that the toll of years of judo has been well worth the price. He wants to share that it is always worthwhile to find the time to take care of your body—and, in his humble opinion, exercise is the best way to do so.

8

RULES FOR THE ENDGAME

I've learned that people will forget what you said, people will forget what you did, but people will never forget how you made them feel.

—Maya Angelou

More people around the world are living longer than ever before, which means it is time to think about how to care for and protect our bodies. Many of us lack guides in life to tell us how to live well. But guideposts and hearing people's stories are important because our goal ought to be not only to survive into old age but also to thrive along the way. This book contains the stories of several people who shared intimate details regarding their perceptions and experiences with aging. I hope my quest to write about *age with agility* illustrates traits that can serve you well as you embrace later stages of life.

Perceptions about aging influenced the way each person featured in this book cared for their body. Connie and Anand, for example, had early life experiences that threatened the promise of long, healthy lives. However, they both hold perceptions of aging that helped them sustain a commitment to maintaining their bodies through movement. In distinct ways, Janice and Max hold complex perceptions of aging shaped by negative role models, but these perceptions also helped motivate them to exercise and care for their bodies in ways that enhanced their daily experience in their later years. Several individuals, including Yvonne, had a concept of aging shaped by having outlived other members of their family. For Yvonne, there is a sense that aging is simply a privilege, and thus there is no need to do much beyond exist with the "extra" time. For others, like Felip, Janice, and Anand, aging is a privilege to be tended to, and they devote time to maintaining their bodies.

Embodied aging can be understood as the ways our environments shape our perceptions about aging and, in turn, the extent to which we maintain or lose functional mobility as we age. Because our interactions with social and physical environments influence our physical and emotional well-being, accounts of personal experiences in later life can help us gain greater understanding of our transitions to mature bodies. Thus, there is great value to listening to, reading, and learning from mature adults about their lived experiences. The stories shared in this book show that there are reasons aging can be associated with slowing down or decline and also that there can be a range of sources of motivation to exercise. Aging is complex, nuanced, and inevitably experienced in different ways by different people. Hearing about different real-life experiences helps us formulate our own rules for the endgame. Each of the people featured in this book illustrated key qualities that include focus, confidence, motivation, resilience, optimism, and commitment. Each person has much to contribute when it comes to caring for our bodies and minds in the long term.

LIVE LONGER, HEALTHIER

In the twenty-first century, we have witnessed the fastest, strongest, and fittest group of mature adults the world has ever seen. At the same time, more of us are spending our time in ways that are sedentary and potentially limiting for our future ability to move. Approximately 80 percent of adults fail to meet basic exercise guidelines, and more than 50 percent of all adults are sedentary for the majority of their day. In many ways, we are living in a world of extremes.[1]

A clear takeaway from interviewing each of these six people over the course of nearly a decade is that, if you do nothing else, try to engage in regular movement in whatever ways you can and seek sustainability so that you can maximize your personal potential over time. Regular exercise is fostered by perceptions of aging that include the idea that aging takes work. Regular bodywork and maintenance should not be considered luxuries or the province of former athletes. It is not essential to have a favorable perception of aging—we have seen in stories like Janice's where negative role models, or observing someone who aged in a way that you want to avoid, can be a powerful motivation, too—however, we must move beyond the idea that aging is necessarily a story of decline.

Gerontology is a field of study that focuses on the experiences and care of mature adults, which teaches us to pay attention to all aspects of the aging process, especially individual lived experiences. There are lessons to learn from those who came before us. It also teaches us that the body inevitably deteriorates with age and that there are things we can do to treat or manage our decline. One important point from the collective experiences shared in this book is that aging with agility has advantages that become even more apparent the longer you live. Another is that aging with agility is not just about physical movement; it is also about mental and emotional adaption to life's challenges, and that all three require regular practice. Developing habits that incorporate time to do squats and to stretch regularly are important, but so is recognizing that agile aging can be associated with being focused, confident, and optimistic in the body you have.

Aging is a story of embracing change and adaptation. Stories about aging hold lessons about how to appreciate the ways that different bodies move and about learning how best to work toward the body that suits your goals. From athletes to regular folks, there are important lessons that each of us can use to shape our own experiences.

Some athletes, particularly elite athletes like Max, possess a competitive drive that serves them well while they are in the game. But once their athletic careers are over and they no longer identify as an athlete, exercise can become anathema. For some, even the *idea* of exercising is a painful reminder of what they once were and will never become again. For those who once inhabited uniquely trained and elite bodies that demonstrated the limits of human potential, intentional movement for the sake of simply being agile later in life can seem like an unworthy goal. This is a challenge for the individual, but it is also a challenge that elite sports and governments around the world ought to consider.

Other former athletes, like Connie and Felipe, built on their athletic experiences as they recalibrated their sense of self in the wake of Olympic glory. Their physical literacy, and possession of the motivation, physical competence, and understanding of the value of engaging in physical movement, helped them pursue other sports and move in ways that kept them agile with age. Both Connie and Felipe, who shared stories of other people they knew who were too extreme in their athletic pursuits, understand that continuing to exercise their bodies is essential to self-preservation. They emphasize the need to find peace with aging in ways that are sustainable.

Janice was never an athlete; in fact, she was actively discouraged from participating in sport in her youth. Yet she is one of the most fit people you will ever meet. Much of her motivation stems from negative role models and her desire to look and feel good. Janice gains confidence by trying not to look or feel her age. She channels her energy and time into exercise because it helps her feel better. Even she admits that she has had many instances of good luck in her life; however, hers is a story about having the confidence to take care of oneself. Even though her early life did not include the development of athletic abilities, she was able to find ways to practice moving, and she has never stopped.

The experiences shared throughout this book contextualize some of the complexities associated with our contemporary collective goal of living longer and healthier. Yvonne demonstrates that it is possible to outlive previous generations even if you never engage in exercise. A potential way to describe Yvonne's route to longevity has been to stay inside and to seek medical attention regularly. Her sedentary behaviors have extremely limited her range of physical mobility, and thus she lives in a sort of conundrum whereby she doesn't move much and thus she can't move much. If and when Yvonne has a bad fall, she relies on public emergency services. She is vulnerable and dependent on her daughter for basic daily activities like toileting. Her life is basically confined to her bed; however, hers is not a life without joy. She maintains a good attitude and a resilient mind.

Anand's story is one that exemplifies the power of each of the chapter headings in this book. Anand was never an athlete, and yet he is the picture of focus, confidence, motivation, resilience, optimism, and commitment. He was told early in life that he would never walk. Decades passed as he struggled to attain basic movement that most people take for granted. Yet he is living a longer healthier life by harnessing the resources he has. Anand is more agile in his seventies than at any other point in his life. Like a true athlete, he has marshalled and created the resources needed to sustain his agility.

Living longer and healthier is a generally acceptable universal goal. It also ought to be universally accepted that there are many ways to move. Anand's story is his own—it's not generalizable. His story is one of privilege and misfortune, of good and bad luck, and of perseverance. His story also illustrates that moving can be a complex endeavor and that there are great benefits to making the effort to move their bodies regularly and intentionally.

This book features a select set of people who have lived on nearly every continent and in very different kinds of bodies. They are unique, and yet they all managed major life challenges and enjoyed certain privileges, including retaining cognitive functioning and avoiding extreme physical limitations, injury, and poverty. They are also individuals who have more time and new chapters ahead.

TIME IS WHAT YOU MAKE OF IT

Just two centuries ago, well under 2 percent of the population was sixty-five years old or older. And now living to at least age sixty-five is a standard expectation in most parts of the world! There are currently over 770 million people age sixty-five and older—that's roughly 10 percent of the planet's population—and demographic trends continue to forecast longevity. Thus, we have to rethink the ways we allocate our time and the time we dedicate to maintaining our bodies. Exercising is not just for athletes, the privileged, the young, or the rich. It is as essential as brushing our teeth. Yet exercise is not something that is universally taught as essential in schools. Exercise might be something a doctor recommends, and some doctors might even write a general exercise prescription, but there is no training in medical school regarding how to help people learn to move their bodies on a regular basis.

Attaining physical literacy and regular engagement in exercise is difficult. Fewer than half of U.S. adults meet the basic physical activity guidelines. The World Health Organization (WHO) reports that physical inactivity is one of the ten leading causes of death in developed countries, despite the fact that modern technology provides an abundance of assistive devices, digital monitors, and equipment that can be used to help us engage in movement to the extent our bodies are able.[2]

The ancient Greeks were advised by Hippocrates that the safest way to be healthy was to exercise regularly and moderately. Many government agencies suggest specific amounts of time that adults should exercise to avoid early death from a sedentary lifestyle. The U.S. Centers for Disease Control and Prevention (CDC) indicates thirty minutes per day, five days a week is optimal. In Japan, the Ministry of Health, Labor, and Welfare indicates that adults should exercise at least 60 minutes every day. Sometimes the prescriptions are not time-bound. The Swedish National Institute of Public Health describes physical activity and exercise as a main health-care objective and advises doctors on how to adapt exercise treatments for individual patients. The American College of Sports Medicine (ACSM) and American Medical Association (AMA) have assessment tools for clinicians to create prescribed exercise routines for adults as a means of rehabilitative care.

We have pursued the desire to live longer, healthier lives for much of human history. For most of that time, however, we have been plagued by infectious disease that cut short this goal. Now we are faced with the plague of chronic disease. As public health attention in the United States and other regions of the world shifts to chronic disease prevention and control, messaging about what it means to be healthy has become both ubiquitous and inconsistent.

As we age, we become more aware of our biological limitations. As a society, we ought to embrace the habit of addressing the challenges associated with developing healthy habits. Our collective goal in aging societies ought to be sustaining functional members of society for as long as possible. And remember that there are many ways to be a member of society. We do not possess the same types of bodies, and our bodies will inevitably change over time. Thus, we need to focus collectively on ways we can be agile.

We can consider several theories from gerontology as we look back on the experiences shared throughout this book. For example, disengagement was proposed in the 1960s as a way of explaining aging as a stage of life in which there is a mutual withdrawal between aging individuals and society. The original idea was based on a study of "normal" aging (which failed to include mature adults with any form of disability or illness) that set out to understand the psyche in adapting to changes associated with aging. Disengagement theory posits that a natural disassociation between aging individuals and society leads to *greater* life satisfaction. Yvonne perhaps illustrates this concept best: she has little engagement with the world beyond her bedroom, yet she feels satisfied with her life. Max, who also maintains lower levels of physical activity and relatively less social engagement, engages in a wider physical domain and indicates that he enjoys the way his time is allocated. Though it has been largely criticized within gerontology, disengagement theory raises a perspective that can help us as consider how we want to spend our time in later chapters of life.[3]

Another prominent theoretical perspective to consider is activity theory, which suggests that quality of life is enhanced by remaining socially and generally active. Here, both Janice and Felipe would score high, while Yvonne would not rank as well. This theory suggests that, as we face loss, for example, because of death among those in our circle or role loss in the case of retirement, we do best to substitute former roles with other activities. Thus, those who pick up hobbies in retirement and meet regularly with others are assumed to do better over time. Here, remaining physically active is favorable, but the central premise is that life satisfaction is tied to remaining engaged and connected with other people. This theory fails to account for important contextual considerations, such as how experiences differ for those who age with substantial physical impairment, how housing matters, and how access to transportation or public infrastructure can act as barriers or facilitators to engaging fully in life in our later years. Living in a city as Yvonne did, where driving is essential, influenced her daily activity levels in adulthood, as did the fact that she never viewed the idea of being socially engaged as connected to her quality of life.[4]

Yet another formative theory that continues to influence current debates about aging is continuity theory, which suggests thinking about ourselves as stable or consistent over time. As we age, we adapt in ways that allow us to feel a sense of continuity with our past selves. Put differently, we evolve in ways that preserve who we are. We maintain our habits, our social and physical environments, and our internal psychological structures. We can observe that Anand maintained a desire to take care of his body and that Connie and Felipe channeled their previous athletic experiences into new exercise habits. Yvonne and Max were also consistent throughout their adulthood in the habits they maintained.[5]

As we consider whether and how to allocate our energy and time toward practicing physical movement, we can evaluate the notion that different ages or stages in life are associated with particular activities and particular levels of engagement. Age stratification theory suggests that age affects the roles individuals play in society and that there are prescriptive activities for people within certain age groups. While the goal of this theory is to understand social patterns, it also imposes an underlying assumption that chronological age can be used to define what we ought to be doing.

But how best to manage our later years? It is well understood that how much money you have impacts how you live, and much has been said about diet and nutrition, what to eat and what to avoid. However, the clearest evidence indicates that regular exercise is the single most important factor under our control when it comes to increasing our chances of living longer and healthier.

THE ATHLETE'S MENTALITY

The athlete's mentality is to be competitive, pursue excellence, and find ways to overcome obstacles to achieve a goal. The athlete's mentality also suggests that we would be well served to focus on the goals and challenges associated with helping all different types of bodies move and engage. This means not only designing and building accessible public spaces but also creating more inclusive programs and supports for people who inhabit different types of bodies. Understanding that there are many types of ideal bodies will help us be more sustainable as individuals and as a society.

Sports are good places to look for this lesson. Sports are incredibly influential in society—we spend billions on them (whether to build new, state-of-the-art facilities; broadcast matches; or buy tickets to see our favorite athletes perform), we set our schedules to watch our favorite sport competitions, and we find our moods deeply affected by their outcomes. We see how completely different types of people and bodies emerge victorious across different sports. And we learn important life skills from sports, from becoming a team player and working toward a collective goal to fostering body confidence and control, becoming accustomed to routine, and even making social change.[6]

However, the life of an elite athlete is one of extremes. One day you are on top of the world; everything comes together and all the practice pays off. The next day, your luck runs dry and your career is over. Even the best players have more losses than wins. The different people represented in this book differed in their associations with athletic experience, but they all had experience with loss and failure. Some channeled their losses into wins—here, I think of Felipe and Anand. Others, like Max, demonstrated that athletic engagement in later adulthood does not always follow patterns started early in life. No longer athletic as a person, Max's world nonetheless revolves around hockey. And Janice was never athletic in her youth but is now in the best shape of her life.

Sports also teach us the importance of high-quality performance over time. The world of competitive sports has fostered many ways of measuring time, length, and quality. It has also fostered an interest in seeing people push themselves to their limits, even at great personal sacrifice. Elite athletes tend to avoid anything near average, instead focusing on their goals, even at the expense of developing a well-rounded, sustainable self. The past couple of decades have demonstrated that the boundaries of what we are physically capable of are moving targets and that the chase for victory has its price. The lived experience for many elite athletes is one of sudden decline, of identity crisis, and of pain.

The experiences of former athletes like Connie, Max, and Felipe illustrate that the rigid focus demanded in elite sports can become a hindrance when it is time to move on. Not one of the three continued to practice the sport to which they devoted the first few chapters of their lives. Connie and Felipe each found new ways of reconnecting with physical movement; Max abandoned all personal engagement in sports and exercise. Their experiences as athletes—and as former athletes—differ, and yet each experienced the power of changing and developing habits over time.

REFLECTIONS ON AGING

Consider that date of birth was not added to the United States census until 1900. In the not-so-distant past, we were much less likely to know our precise ages. Each person I interviewed had different ideas about how their perceptions of aging affected their experience of aging, as well as the exercise habits they maintained or failed to maintain. Each reflected on how their bodies had changed over time—sometimes in ways they saw as good, and sometimes in ways they understood as bad. Some felt younger with each passing year. It is important to remember that age tends to hold the meaning we give it.[7] The way you operate your body in your later years depends on how you operationalize the construct of time; the extent to which you allocate your time to intentional physical movement; and ultimately on the extent to which we, as individuals and as a society, embrace aging. It comes down to developing agility.

But what does it mean to live in an aging body? The oxidative stress theory of aging suggests that oxidative stress occurs from imbalances that interact with the naturally occurring loss of tissue and organ functioning that takes place over time. Oxidation is why some fruits get dark spots and turn brown. It is also why our skin gets brown spots and why it loses collagen and elastin fibers, resulting in variegation, wrinkles, and sagging.

Billions of dollars are made because we buy antiaging products that aim to minimize the signs of oxidation. Depictions of aging as a time of decline, decay, and decrepitude can change our perceptions of what it means to be in an aging body. Not only does the sense that natural aging is to be avoided prompt reactions of disgust and distrust, but it can also prompt the desire to avoid spending time with people who display the signs of it.[8]

One of the underlying messages in this book, however, is that being healthy and fit looks different in different bodies. Connie and Janice each illustrate high levels of functional mobility, and yet sharp contrasts are evident when you consider the differences in their athletic backgrounds. There are also contrasts when you consider Janice's use of facial injections, hair dyes, and cosmetic surgery and Connie's natural look. Each has the face and body of a person who has successfully reached advanced age, although they may look very different on the surface.

It is also true that motivations and sources of inspiration to exercise and stay fit vary. Whereas Max lost his personal commitment to exercise once he stopped being an athlete, Felipe adapted and found a new sport. For Janice and Felipe, the quest to attain more youthful versions of beauty served as powerful motivators. For Anand and Connie, the quest to keep their bodies moving was a powerful incentive. As Anand and his partner, Myrna, demonstrate, there are many important ways to keep agile and functionally mobile. In their own ways, Felipe, Anand, Max, Connie, and Janice all described exercise or sport as a religion at various times in their life.

The lived experience of, relationship to, and understandings of exercise for the rest of the group provides a sharp contrast to Yvonne, who has found herself physically limited and immobile because of lack of movement. For both Yvonne and Max, there are concerns about exercise that are linked to fears of getting their heart rate too high. Each was concerned that exercise is risky. Max developed a strong and unfortunate understanding of exercise as being only for "athletes." And he linked being an athlete with elite abilities and high performance sport. The failure of both Yvonne and Max to have more holistic understandings of exercise ultimately contributed to their limited physical functional abilities.

There are many ways to think about and experience our final decades. The extent to which we fight or give in to the passing of time depends on the extent to which we fear or embrace aging. An ongoing challenge is how to manage our individual and societal obsessions with youth and speed while acknowledging our collective need to embrace aging.

CHANGE YOUR HABITS, CHANGE YOUR LIFE

Aging is about developing habits or acquiring behaviors that become routine. Regular smoking is a bad habit; daily exercise is a good habit. Habits occur regularly and are formed by behavioral and neurological patterns. But developing favorable habits can be difficult. They can take time to learn, and they often require extensive practice. Where possible, we should try to acclimate and get comfortable with a good habit so that something like exercise, which might have once seemed foreign or was practiced intermittently, becomes habitual.

The hard part for many of us is finding the motivation to engage in a good behavior long enough to make it a habit. The people who shared their stories in this book show us that habits can be shaped by positive and negative sources of inspiration. A great deal of attention is paid to heroes in sport, but the power of a negative role model should not be underestimated. Janice described a desire to avoid aging like her mother, and Max discussed a desire to avoid being like his father and other negative influences in his life. Yvonne serves in some ways as a model to avoid—even for her daughter Maria. It is important to remember, however, that Yvonne doesn't see herself as a negative role model. She views herself as resilient, and her ability to endure and remain in good spirits is a testament to that.

Connie's experience shows that some people do well by forming exercise habits that break their routines into chunks, forming small movement goals on the path to larger ones. Felipe, on the other hand, demonstrates how some do well by forming exercise habits that find a source of inspiration and using that inspiration to hold themselves accountable. Felipe, like Janice, also highlights the challenges associated with an orientation toward aging that is focused on trying to age without showing signs of aging.

Every habit starts with a cue that tells your brain to do a certain action. This is followed by the behavior and then a reward, which helps your brain remember that it wants to make the decision to repeat this behavior. Behavior becomes a habit when you don't have to think hard about making the decision to engage in the behavior. As a person living with disability and as an economist, Anand consistently shared his belief that time spent exercising was the most optimal use of his time. Connie and Felipe both shared stories of athletes who pushed themselves to the limit so that their bodies became less functional. Janice commented on her luck in life and demonstrated that operating without any major injuries is an enormous privilege. In addition, her dedication to regular movement can be contrasted with Yvonne, who lived a life free of major injury and yet avoided engagement in almost all forms of physical movement.

Many healthy or desirable behaviors feel uncomfortable at first. They don't often come with immediate rewards. Anand, for instance, shows that it can take decades to feel the progress from exercising. And his experience suggests that forming certain new habits should feel uncomfortable. Starting a new jogging habit is likely to feel difficult, and a weight-lifting routine is likely to leave you sore; both are even harder if you already have pain, fatigue, and other limiting factors.

Evidence from the stories shared in this book also illustrates that major disruptions in our routines provide opportunities to create new routines. New routines can include substance abuse, as in the case with Max, who shifted from being a high-performance athlete to being an addict. Or disruptions to old routines may reignite the desire to enhance functional abilities, as in the case of Anand, who has found himself getting stronger with each move he makes in life. Connie and Felipe each made the choice to get on more sustainable paths and maintain engagement in physical activities when their elite athletic careers ended. Even small changes in our environment, for example, when we move, go on vacation, or hit a milestone birthday, can present opportunities to change our habits because they change our cues and potentially alter the rewards we perceive.

When we make time to develop habits, we eventually develop the ability to perform behaviors with greater ease. All the people in this book illustrate that the choice to allocate time to moving the body and flexing the mind is a decision well made.

GUIDELINES FROM THE INTERVIEWEES

Adulthood is a time for codes. Without them, we are locked out from the experiences we seek and those we have worked to create. Aging is about learning how to live in the spaces you create for yourself and how to protect what you have. Aging with agility is learning to live in your body using the codes that help you sustain habits to maintain your body. As you formulate your own rules for the endgame, consider the following advice shared by the people featured in this book.

PAY ATTENTION TO THE RESOURCES YOU NEED AND THE RESOURCES YOU HAVE TO GIVE

My advice is that the sooner you can figure out the resources you need and how to get them, the better off you are going to be. Keep in mind that you are going to need to give, too. You will feel better when you give, but it might not always be an even exchange. Pay attention as if your life depended on it—this is important in school, at work. Pay attention to your children, and pay attention to not fall down. Always best if you can focus on what you are doing; let yourself feel content with that, be ready to share what you are good at, and then don't be afraid to figure out the resources you need.

—CONNIE

JUST MOVE

If you are feeling meh, get up and move. If you are feeling pain, use that to motivate yourself and move around. If it's anxiety, then use that energy to go for a walk. If you are feeling that you want to slim down, go for a walk. If you are tired, get up and do some movement. Just move. Use whatever it is that is bothering you or whatever works for you to keep moving. Don't say, "I'll do it tomorrow." Who knows if there's tomorrow? There is today, and today will not be wasted if you do some moving.

—JANICE

TAKE CARE OF YOUR BODY LIKE YOU'RE GONNA NEED IT FOR A LONG TIME

Don't be like me. Being truly competitive means playing through to the end. Look, you should always keep your eyes on the prize, go for the goal, and remember being mentally ready is as important as physically ready. I guess, most of all, I would say take care of your body like your gonna need it for a long time. Never thought I was gonna be around this long. I might have done things, yeah, I would have done things differently if I really ever thought I'd make it this long.

—MAX

ENJOY LIFE MORE

Nobody is on their deathbed wishing they worked more. I heard that on TV the other day. I'm sure that's true. People regret more working on things they didn't feel good about. I lay here, and I wish I did more things to enjoy life more. Don't lie in bed wishing you did more. My advice is enjoy—and take the risks you need to so you can enjoy life more.

—YVONNE

DO NOT FEAR WHAT COMES NEXT

I don't like it when people give me advice, a lot of it has proven wrong, but I'll humor you here. I will say, don't focus on fear and do not fear what comes next. You do not know that what will come next will be worse. There are no special prizes for fearing the worst. Look at me, my life has only gotten better. I suspect it will continue to do so.

—ANAND

BRUSH YOUR TEETH AND LEARN HOW TO FALL

First, I would advise people to brush your teeth. Like me, I wasn't always taking the best care, then I was brushing too hard, lots of receding. So I said, "Okay, I'm going to start brushing with my left hand." So I have this daily task and now don't brush so hard. So I would say, "Brush, okay? No excuses." Also, learn how to fall. This is important. In judo, we practice this; in life, most people don't. Learning how to fall is probably the most important thing, though.

—FELIPE

AGILE AGING

Greater longevity for the masses, or having more people live longer on average, has enormous implications for all aspects of life and society. We are always in between the past and what comes next. We all have an expiration date. The bodies we inhabit in the liminal space that comes between birth and death is a function of the bodies we are born into, how we experience the world with these bodies, and how we take care of them. It is my hope that the stories shared throughout these pages will help you reflect on the time you have and make use of it in ways that help you maintain an agile, sustainable presence.

The quote by Maya Angelou at the start of this chapter suggests that people forget many things, but they never forget how you made them feel. In many ways, this sums up the goal of this project, which is to evoke feelings in you about how you want to carry out your life in relation to intentional physical movement. People who love exercise usually claim it makes them feel great. People who don't exercise often don't like being made to think about it. I hope that listening to how others think about it, over time and from a range of different orientations, will evoke an interest that changes how you relate to movement.

When Anand, Janice, Connie, and Felipe talk about exercising as something they do, they understand exercise as connected to their core life purpose. Max had other interests and a different sense of purpose in his life. Yvonne struggled to exercise throughout her life, in part because she never connected it to her sense of self.

Each of us comes to appreciate life and understand our own aging as a process controlled by both fate and free will. Some of us are lucky enough to avoid major illness and injury; others are clever enough to find our own ways to develop meaningful ideas about what it means to age successfully. For some people, aging is something to fight because advanced age is associated with decreased desirability. Others age strategically so we can avoid rigid understandings of aging and the restrictive norms society imposes about how we ought to look and act at a certain age.

We all search for and find meaning in life in different ways. Today, many of us will have longer than ever to find meaning and carve out our own ways to live and thrive—to age with agility.

METHODOLOGICAL APPENDIX

This appendix is meant to give you an understanding of how I embarked on, documented, examined, analyzed, and compiled the adventure that is the basis of this book. I use the word "adventure" to describe the process of writing this book because what started as a short-term project turned into an approximately decade-long inquiry into the lives of people as they embraced mature adulthood and talked with me about their exercise habits.

I began the project with the hypothesis that elite athletes would have insights into how to sustain exercise routines well into mature adulthood. I learned quickly that they did but that their insights were not straightforward. Life experience influences our bodies in many ways, and so I shifted away from an exclusive focus on athletes. My goal became studying the meaning and motivations people in later stages of life attributed to exercise and understanding whether and how their perceptions about aging influenced their exercise habits. This required that I look at individuals' accounts of their own life courses rather than employing theoretical concepts or biological markers discretely. Like many researchers before me, my method was to gather data on people's lives and to explore how people interpreted their experiences. What emerged was a series of stories that I tried to unpack and learn from.[1]

During early interviews, I often shared meals or snacks with participants. Some of us walked and even did exercise classes together. Discussions sometimes arose about participants' eating habits or specific exercise regimens. Food, diet, specific types of exercises, and a few other topics arose occasionally, but these topics were not featured in this book because they were not discussed consistently across all participants and because they were not the intended focus of this book. This book is about people's relationships to their bodies, and much has been written elsewhere about how to maintain a specific body through specific exercises, diets, and so on. Here, I have chosen to focus broadly on movement to underscore the many potential ways for different bodies (and minds) to become and be agile.

I chose to focus on movement among people who moved in different ways. However, I did not capture anything generalizable as it relates to being a person navigating accessibility challenges and/or with disability. Many of the participants I interviewed experienced significant mobility issues, access challenges, and chronic disease, including chronic pain, depression, diabetes, undiagnosed ailments, and polio, to name a few. These issues were unique experiences for the participants and, in some cases, were described as key motivators for regular engagement in exercise. I make this note about the varying levels of ability and disability that arose throughout this book to clarify that these experiences are nuanced, complex, and affect individuals in different ways.

This sample is also unique because it features people who were willing to engage and share their stories. They hail from several different regions of the world, but one thing they all had in common was being over sixty-five years old at the start of my study. This is a point in life when many people traditionally stopped working, which can mean having more time on their hands. And for some people, it can be a phase of life where there is more time for exercise and body maintenance. Despite the fact that most of the people who shared their stories with me enjoyed relatively good health at the point I interviewed them, there were several occasions when we talked about death, and this was perhaps because of the participants' stage in life or because a global pandemic (one that disproportionately killed older people) occurred in the midst of data collection. While this book is about later chapters in life, it was by no means intended to focus on people's *last* chapters. Thus, I spent relatively little time writing here about participants' reflections on death or dying.[2]

I do not know how long each person I interviewed will continue to live; I do not know when or how their stories will end. Therefore, these in-depth interviews inherently generated incomplete knowledge. I am confident that the stories included here contribute to our understanding of the later stages in life in meaningful ways. I must acknowledge, however, that these are the stories of people who are continuing their life story, the stories of people who demonstrate persistence and resiliency. They have lived many years on this planet, and they may have many, many more years and stories ahead of them.[3]

METHODOLOGY

Qualitative research is an interpretative, naturalistic approach to understanding the meaning people bring to understanding different phenomena, beginning with the assumption that these meanings matter. Constructivism asserts that individuals' perceptions of their experiences are constructed from their reflections on those experiences. The approach I used here also includes an implicit assumption of multiple, subjective realities. It allows for unresolved contradictions within and across data.

My research goal was to examine perceptions about exercise and aging from a unique set of mature people. My intention has never been to make broad, sweeping generalizations about exercise or, for that matter, mature adults. Thus, an iterative, narrative approach provided an ideal framework for collecting, analyzing, and interpreting lived experience.[4]

The field of gerontology emphasizes perceptions about life from the standpoint of those *in* later life. Narrative gerontology encourages the researcher to listen, discuss substantive issues, and engage with people on multiple occasions. Experience is valued, and life stories are understood not as exact replicas of events that have transpired but as narratives that weave together perceptions and interpretations of the individual's experience. The approach is intuitive and explicitly assumes that the primary way humans make meaning of experiences is by sharing stories. Guided by this methodological approach, I used qualitative interviews to generate each person's perceptions of their body over time and the nature of their relationship with exercise. Narrative gerontology, the life-course perspective, and embodied aging informed my approach to this book.[5]

The life-course perspective has been used to suggest that people process normative expectations of age in the context of their own circumstances. Life stories are ways that people describe what they think is most meaningful about their own lives. According to this perspective, early experiences may affect life-course trajectories and later-life transitions. The key principles of the life-course perspective include developmental timing, historical time and place, human agency, and linked lives. For developmental timing, the life-course perspective suggests that people make plans and decisions that are shaped by their own personal histories and social circumstances. This means that exposure to exercise or sports earlier in life may influence behavior patterns later in life. It implies that perceptions about aging are shaped by favorable as well as unfavorable experiences and exposures earlier in life. Developmental timing matters because humans develop in biologically, socially, and psychologically meaningful ways over the life course that influence behavioral habits and routines.[6]

The second principle, historical time and place, states that expectations emerge not only out of individual experience but also out of interactions with broad economic and cultural expectations that reflect the historical time and place in which they occur. Nearly all my study participants grew up around the time of the Great Depression or started in life without great financial wealth. This affected their sense of determination, perceptions about exercise, and understanding of how best to take care of their bodies. Notwithstanding the importance of sociohistorical factors, people retain a level of human agency—the third principle recognized in life-course research—that allows them to make choices that adapt or react to their context. Several participants reflected on feeling or not feeling regret over the choices they made in life. This sense of agency changed over time and guided their later-life reflections regarding their relationships to health and acceptance of their bodies.

The fourth principle looks at how the degree to which lives are linked can influence a person's experiences and transitions into and out of each stage of the life course. This last principle influenced the development of this book as participants discussed their spouses, or their life partners popped into online video chats or joined us at interviews. In the case of every participant except Max, another person entered the interviews over the years: Connie's husband Ken, Janice's friend Tina, Yvonne's daughter Maria, Anand's life partner Myrna, and Felipe's husband Alex. Each shed light on the person featured in ways that enhanced my understanding about their values and their perceptions about aging. They helped me better understand each interviewee's priorities about exercise.

This book takes a phenomenological approach to thinking about senescence, or the process of growing old. It gives embodiment to, or the representation or realization of, how interactions with social and physical environments influence our physical, psychological, and emotional well-being, an important place in understanding what it is like to transition into mature adulthood. By focusing on the perspectives of a set of people who were born into very different types of bodies, from elite athletes to people living with physical limitations, this book approaches aging as an experience that inherently centers around the dynamics of the body. Embodiment can be understood as the ways that bodily processes are intertwined with and shaped by social processes.

Corporeality, or the fact of existing as a physical body, can be understood in the context of aging and embodiment as reflective of the social contexts in which we live and the cultural beliefs we hear, learn, and incorporate about aging. I make no claims about the optimal body type or the ideal way to move your body. I do claim that engagement in physical movement changes over time and is influenced by biological and social processes as well as adoptive and individual factors. Epigenetics is the influence of one's environment on their gene expression, and embodied aging aims to understand the ways our environment shapes our perceptions about aging and in turn how we age. The approach I took here aimed to longitudinally explore ways perceptions about aging shape attitudes and engagement in exercise.

METHODS

My primary method of data collection was in-depth, semis-tructured interviews. I took a narrative approach that allowed participants to situate their responses within the context they believed most appropriate to their story. The names of all partici-pants and family members are pseudonyms, and I have changed some identifying characteristics to protect the confidentiality of all individuals, as promised in the informed consent process. My first formal interviews began in 2012, when I worked with a set of community organizations, senior centers, and targeted social organizations. I also connected with some participants who had been elite athletes and coaches through another project I was conducting about athletic retirement.[7]

Interview Style and Setting

My interviews had a conversational style. I inquired about participants' experiences, habits, and perceptions of exercise; their motivation to exercise or to avoid it; and their thoughts about aging and mature adulthood, including any role models or people in their lives who they sought to emulate or avoid being like. My interview guide was also designed from the life-course theoretical perspective. Thus, I asked participants to tell me about their childhoods, including where they grew up and their exposures to sport and exercise as a child. The order of the questions varied across participants, and many of the questions, such as those about exercise habits, were repeated over their life course and over the years in which our repeated interviews took place. Although I had a fair number of questions and probes, my goal was always to speak as little as possible.

Most of my interviews took place in Canada and the United States; some took place in Germany and Japan. Some interviews were held in a coffee shop or other neutral setting. Many interviews took place over the phone or through an online video platform. Most interviews were audio recorded and transcribed verbatim. I also took notes during the interviews and immediately afterward to capture additional data.

The interviews took place in person and online over a relatively long and unique period. This allowed me to observe changes in each person: sometimes we were pulled into different directions (for example, when we checked in with each other during the early months of the pandemic). Thus, we did not follow a linear process. We sometimes focused on the present; sometimes we jumped to the past and mused about the future.

Analysis of the Data

My analytic process included listening to audio recordings of my interviews, reading transcribed interviews, and reviewing my notes repeatedly. After I familiarized myself with the interviews, I coded each transcript. I began with an open-ended code sheet in which I created initial ("first-level") codes that corresponded to responses to questions I had asked each participant over the course of approximately twenty interviews per person. I conducted a second round of coding in which I formed categories for each person based on their life stories, which later turned into relevant themes. I worked with some participants to frame their stories in chronological order; with others, I followed a flow that was more erratic but suited their personality or general style. The patterns that emerged were based firmly on descriptions provided by participants. Whenever possible, I included quotes that pertained to a particular theme or helped elucidate the individual's experience.[8]

Notes on Interviewing Participants Through the Pandemic

It is worth commenting on the implications of having conducted interviews before, during, and after the COVID-19 pandemic. Since the turn of the twenty-first century until just before the pandemic in 2020, life expectancy had been on an upward trajectory around the world. When I first started this project, much was being written about this remarkable upward trajectory and the implications of a longer life. During the COVID-19 pandemic, life expectancy for adults sixty years old and over dropped for the first time in approximately seventy years.

While the pandemic threw a wrench into many people's lives and in life expectancy patterns, it also allowed me to connect with participants on a different level. The uncertainty we shared in the early days led us to share candid, off-script concerns. Every participant included in this book lost a friend or family member in the pandemic. One participant I hoped to include in the book died during the pandemic, and their story is not shared. Each participant and I compared notes on how protocols and reactions varied around the world. I shared some details about my life and concerns with participants during our calls and was generally much less inhibited or private than I might have been in the past. In retrospect, I believe this new shared experience opened our conversations in ways that allowed for greater insights and reflections.

REFLECTIONS AS THE INTERVIEWER

What is presented in this book is inherently subject to my interpretation. My perceptions about the concepts of fitness and exercise are biased by my experiences and my position in the life course. Exercise is always an effort. Perhaps because I am almost entirely unathletic, I am fascinated by those who are. When I listen to people who move their bodies in ways that would be impossible for me, both physically and mentally, I instinctively want to know more.

It is important for me not only to highlight my own bias as an outsider to the world of sport and athletics but also to acknowledge the privilege and honor that comes with interviewing people at later stages in the life course. Talking with people who are older than me is something I have always cherished. My mother tells me that, as a child, I would pretend to play with the children, but she could tell I was always more interested in listening in on the parents' conversations.

A FINAL PERSONAL NOTE

After I submitted my first full version of this manuscript to the press, I developed a very painful case of shingles. Because I was unfamiliar with its symptoms, I assumed I had somehow hurt myself from a recent attempt to exercise and had burned myself from the heating pad I was using to ease the pain. In any event, I missed the treatment window, and the pain became more excruciating than my experiences with giving birth. In the aftermath, I questioned what right I had to write a book about exercise and aging when some people deal with pain and limitations that make exercise seem like an absurd proposition.

As I recovered, I had a phone call with Yvonne in which I mentioned the shingles. She conveyed her sympathy and pointed out that my being an "active" person probably helped my recovery. While I might have expected this insight to have come from Janice, getting it from Yvonne helped me realize two things. One, I didn't recover as quickly or as easily as I would have liked, and I needed to use my experiences to motivate myself to become more agile in my own understandings of movement with age. Two, and perhaps more important, she helped me realize that there is always more to a person than you think.

Although my interviews spanned approximately a decade, they capture only a snapshot of participants' experiences. It has been said before: the interviewer never quite knows how the story will end. I hope that you find what is shared here meaningful in ways that help you navigate your own path to agility.[9]

NOTES

1. ON YOUR MARK

1. Please see the methodological appendix for more information on the methods and approach I employed as I conducted the interviews that are at the heart of this book.

2. For more on embodiment and its applications within gerontology, see, for example, Mike Featherstone and Mike Hepworth, "Ageing, the Life Course and the Sociology of Embodiment," in *Modernity, Medicine and Health*, ed. Graham Scambler and Paul Higgs (Routledge, 1998), 147–75. See also Stephen Katz, "Hold On! Falling, Embodiment, and the Materiality of Old Age," in *Corpus: An Interdisciplinary Reader on Bodies and Knowledge*, ed. Monica J. Casper and Paisley Currah (Palgrave Macmillan US, 2011), 187–205. For more on epigenetics, see Christina Pagiatakis, Elettra Musolino, Rosalba Gornati, Giovanni Bernardini, and Roberto Papait, "Epigenetics of Aging and Disease: A Brief Overview," *Aging Clinical and Experimental Research* 33 (2021): 737–45.

3. World Health Organization, *Constitution of the World Health Organization* (World Health Organization, 1946), https://www.who.int/about /governance/constitution.

4. Scholars have employed a range of definitions of health over time and different ways of examining health and exercise. See, for example, John M. Jakicic, William E. Kraus, Kenneth E. Powell et al., "Association Between Bout Duration of Physical Activity and Health: Systematic Review," *Medicine and Science in Sports and Exercise* 51, no. 6 (2019): 1213–19.

See also Fiona C. Bull, Salih S. Al-Ansari, Stuart Biddle et al., "World Health Organization 2020 Guidelines on Physical Activity and Sedentary Behaviour," *British Journal of Sports Medicine* 54, no. 24 (2020): 1451–62; World Health Organization, *Constitution of the World Health Organization*. And for an interesting review of the literature examining health and purpose or meaning in life, see Katarzyna Czekierda, Anna Banik, Crystal L. Park, and Aleksandra Luszczynska, "Meaning in Life and Physical Health: Systematic Review and Meta-Analysis," *Health Psychology Review* 11, no. 4 (2017): 387–418.

5. See Phillip Hancock, Bill Hughes, Elizabeth Jagger et al., *The Body, Culture and Society: An Introduction* (Open University, 2000). See also Emanuelle Tulle-Winton, "Growing Old and Resistance: Towards a New Cultural Economy of Old," *Ageing & Society* 19, no. 3 (1999): 281–99.

6. For more on early literary and cinematic depictions of older adults, see Andrea Charise, *The Aesthetics of Senescence: Aging, Population, and the Nineteenth-Century British Novel* (State University of New York Press, 2020); Cynthia Miller and Bowdoin Van Riper, *Elder Horror: Essays on Film's Frightening Images of Aging* (McFarland, 2019); Timothy Shary and Nancy McVittie, *Fade to Gray: Aging in American Cinema* (University of Texas Press, 2016).

7. For more on the medicalized body, see Michel Foucalt, *The Birth of the Clinic* (Parthenon, 1973). For thoughtful critiques of the medicalized body, see also Stephen Katz, *Cultural Aging: Life Course, Lifestyle, and Senior Worlds* (University of Toronto Press, 2005).

8. For more on the media's treatment of women and ways the media aims to manipulate women's bodies, see Renne Engeln, *Beauty Sick: How the Cultural Obsession with Appearance Hurts Girls and Women* (HarperCollins, 2017).

9. Among many of Emmanuelle Tulle-Winton's insightful works on the topic of aging bodies is an excellent book about sports participation later in life and aging embodiment. See Emmanuelle Tulle, *Ageing, the Body and Social Change: Running in Later Life* (Springer, 2008).

10. For a research-based approach to examining social determinants of health and exercise with age, see, for example, Alana Diniz Cavalcanti, Rafael da Silveira Moreira, George Tadeu Nunes Diniz, Mirella

Bezerra Rodrigues Vilela, and Vanessa de Lima Silva, "Active Aging and Its Interface with Social Determinants of Health," *Geriatrics, Gerontology and Aging* 12, no. 1 (2018): 15–23.

11. Systematic reviews are considered the gold standard in research because they attempt to identify, synthesize, and appraise all the empirical evidence on a given topic. There have been numerous systematic reviews documenting the benefits of exercise on the aging body. See, for example, Cathie Sherrington, Nicola Fairhall, Geraldine Wallbank et al., "Exercise for Preventing Falls in Older People Living in the Community: An Abridged Cochrane Systematic Review," *British Journal of Sports Medicine* 54, no. 15 (2020): 885–91. See also Feng-Tzu Chen, Jennifer L. Etnier, Kuei-Hui Chan, Ping-Kun Chiu, Tsung-Ming Hung, and Yu-Kai Chang, "Effects of Exercise Training Interventions on Executive Function in Older Adults: A Systematic Review and Meta-Analysis," *Sports Medicine* 50, no. 8 (2020): 1451–67; Ryan S. Falck, Jennifer C. Davis, John R. Best, Rachel A. Crockett, and Teresa Liu-Ambrose, "Impact of Exercise Training on Physical and Cognitive Function Among Older Adults: A Systematic Review and Meta-Analysis," *Neurobiology of Aging* 79 (2019): 119–30.

12. Francis A. Albert, Melissa J. Crowe, Aduli E. O. Malau-Aduli, and Bunmi S. Malau-Aduli, "Physical Activity Promotion: A Systematic Review of the Perceptions of Healthcare Professionals," *International Journal of Environmental Research and Public Health* 17, no. 12 (2020): 4358–94.

13. Colleen Tully-Wilson, Richard Bojack, Prudence M. Millear, Helen M. Stallman, Andrew Allen, and Jonathan Mason, "Self-Perceptions of Aging: A Systematic Review of Longitudinal Studies," *Psychology and Aging* 36, no. 7 (2021): 773–89. See also Simone Hausknecht, Lee-Fay Low, Kate O'Loughlin, Justin McNab, and Lindy Clemson, "Older Adults' Self-Perceptions of Aging and Being Older: A Scoping Review," *Gerontologist* 60, no. 7 (2020): 524–34.

14. Among the many books within the rich literature on healthy aging, I recommend Peter Attia and Bill Gifford, *Outlive: The Science and Art of Longevity* (Harmony, 2023). See also Peter Attia's highly engaging podcast *Drive*. See also David A. Sinclair and Matthew D. LaPlante, *Lifespan: Why We Age—and Why We Don't Have To* (Atria, 2019).

15. See, for example, Charles A. Popkin, Ahmad F. Bayomy, and Christopher S. Ahmad, "Early Sport Specialization," *Journal of the American Academy of Orthopaedic Surgeons* 27, no. 22 (2019): e995–e1000.

16. Mark Hamer, Richard Weiler, and Emmanuel Stamatakis, "Watching Sport on Television, Physical Activity, and Risk of Obesity in Older Adults," *BMC Public Health* 14, no. 1 (2014): 1–4.

17. For a great read on an amazing master athlete see Bruce Grierson, *What Makes Olga Run? The Mystery of the 90-Something Track Star and What She Can Teach Us About Living Longer, Happier Lives* (Macmillan, 2014). See also Gregory A. Tayrose, Bryan G. Beutel, Dennis A. Cardone, and Orrin H. Sherman, "The Master Athlete: A Review of Current Exercise and Treatment Recommendations," *Sports Health* 7, no. 3 (2015): 270–76.

18. Maximal oxygen consumption has been used by the American Heart Association to assess risk of cardiovascular disease as well as a measure to validate physical activity guidelines.

19. For notable works on the history of exercise see Daniel Lieberman, *Exercised: The Science of Physical Activity, Rest, and Health* (Penguin UK, 2020). See also Bill Hayes, *Sweat: A History of Exercise* (Bloomsbury, 2022); Alex Hutchinson, *Endure: Mind, Body, and the Curiously Elastic Limits of Human Performance* (HarperCollins, 2018).

20. The first physical education textbook was published in 1800, titled *Gymnastik für die Jugend* (*Gymnastics for the Youth*), it became a standard reference for physical education.

21. For more detail on the risks of sitting and other sedentary behaviors, see Aviroop Biswas, Paul I. Oh, Guy E. Faulkner et al., "Sedentary Time and Its Association with Risk for Disease Incidence, Mortality, and Hospitalization in Adults: A Systematic Review and Meta-Analysis," *Annals of Internal Medicine* 162, no. 2 (2015): 123–32.

22. Demographic transitions are changes in population dynamics within a country as it moves from having a high fertility rate and high mortality rate to low fertility and low mortality rates.

23. Important work has demonstrated through systematic reviews of the literature the links between and risks of being sedentary and chronic health conditions. See, for example, Renqing Zhao, Wenqian Bu, Yingfeng Chen, and Xianghe Chen, "The Dose-Response Associations of Sedentary Time with Chronic Diseases and the Risk for

All-Cause Mortality Affected by Different Health Status: A Systematic Review and Meta-Analysis," *Journal of Nutrition, Health & Aging* 24, no. 1 (2020): 63–70.

24. For a detailed perspective on the intersections between race, gender, and aging see Arline T. Geronimus, *Weathering: The Extraordinary Stress of Ordinary Life in an Unjust Society* (Hachette, 2023).

25. Laura Hurd Clarke, "Women, Aging, and Beauty Culture: Navigating the Social Perils of Looking Old," *Generations* 41, no. 4 (2018): 104–8. See also Rebecca Bassett-Gunter, Desmond McEwan, and Aria Kamarhie, "Physical Activity and Body Image Among Men and Boys: A Meta-Analysis," *Body Image* 22 (2017): 114–28.

26. See the methodological appendix for more detail.

2. FOCUS

1. Until late in the twentieth century, an athlete who represented their country in the Olympic Games had to be an amateur athlete; anyone considered professional or who earned money from their sport was banned from competition. An iconic turning point in the Olympics that defines the leap from amateur to allowing professional athletes took place at the Barcelona Games in 1992, when some of the most famous players from the National Basketball Association (NBA) participated on the so-called U.S. Dream Team. Today professional athletes can compete in an Olympic Games alongside amateur athletes, although boxing and wrestling discourage professionals.

2. For a review of the literature, see Danielle A. N. Chapa, Sarah N. Johnson, Brianne N. Richson et al., "Eating-Disorder Psychopathology in Female Athletes and Non-Athletes: A Meta-Analysis," *International Journal of Eating Disorders* 55, no. 7 (2022): 861–85.

3. See, for example, Lisa Rotenstein, MatthewTorre, Marcos Ramos et al., "Prevalence of Burnout Among Physicians: A Systematic Review," *JAMA* 320, no. 11 (2018): 1131–50.

4. In the late 1950s and 1960s, elite female gymnasts were typically 5 feet, 5 inches tall, while today the average height for a female gymnast is under 5 feet because there are advantages to being small for the types of routines gymnasts are now evaluated for. Nadia Comaneci introduced the double back flip, something most people thought of as impossible,

to the 1976 Olympics, and she is credited with shifting the trend toward smaller, more powerful gymnasts.

5. In many ways, this experience reflects elements of post-traumatic stress disorder (PTSD), a mental health condition caused by extremely stressful events. For more on mental health issues that can be relevant in elite sports, see Carsten Larsen, Karin Moesch, Natalie Durand-Bush, and Kristoffer Henriksen, *Mental Health in Elite Sport: Applied Perspectives from Across the Globe* (Routledge, 2021).

3. CONFIDENCE

1. Ben Cosgrove, "The Luckiest Generation: LIFE with Teenagers in 1950s America," *Time*, November 29, 2014, https://time.com/3544391/the-luckiest-generation-life-with-teenagers-in-1950s-america/.

2. Susan Ware, *Homeward Bound: American Families in the Cold War Era* (Basic Books, 1988).

3. In the United States, the 1940s saw the largest proportional rise in women's workforce participation of the entire twentieth century.

4. For interesting reads on sex and romantic love in later adulthood, see, for example, Joan Price, *Naked at Our Age: Talking Out Loud About Senior Sex* (Seal Press, 2011); Carol Denker, *Autumn Romance: Stories and Portraits of Love After 50* (A-Shirley, 2020); Beth Montemurro and Jenna Marie Siefken, "Cougars on the Prowl? New Perceptions of Older Women's Sexuality," *Journal of Aging Studies* 28 (2014): 35–43; Sara Arber, Kate Davidson, and Jay Ginn, *Gender and Ageing: Changing Roles and Relationships* (McGraw-Hill Education, 2003).

5. Critical gerontology has articulated thoughtful criticisms of consumer marketing, often disguised as health promotion, pressuring us to fight aging by any means. See, for example, Stephen Katz and Barbara Marshall, "New Sex for Old: Lifestyle, Consumerism, and the Ethics of Aging Well," *Journal of Aging Studies* 17, no. 1 (2003): 3–16; Barbara Marshall, "'Hard Science': Gendered Constructions of Sexual Dysfunction in the 'Viagra Age,'" *Sexualities* 5, no. 2 (2002): 131–58.

6. See Clare Anderson, "Menopause and the 'Menoboom': How Older Women Are Desexualised by Culture," in *Desexualisation in Later Life: The Limits of Sex and Intimacy*, ed. Paul Simpson, Paul Reynolds, and Trish Hafford-Letchfield (Policy Press, 2021), 77–94.

7. John W. Rowe and Robert L. Kahn, "Human Aging: Usual and Successful," *Science* 237 (1987): 143–49. See also John W. Rowe and Robert L. Kahn, "Successful Aging," *Gerontologist* 37 (1997): 433–40; John W. Rowe and Robert L. Kahn, *Successful Aging* (Pantheon/Random House, 1998).

8. For an overview of critical perspectives on successful aging, with numerous references for more insight, see Stephen Katz and Toni Calasanti, "Critical Perspectives on Successful Aging: Does It Appeal More Than It Illuminates?," *Gerontologist* 55, no. 1 (2015): 26–33.

9. Evidence suggests that most adults actually feel younger than their chronological age by around eight years, starting as they approach their thirties. This is helpful because another body of evidence suggests that positive perceptions of aging correspond to better health outcomes, including living longer. In other words, you are only as old as you feel, and most of us feel pretty young. For a review of this literature, see Simone Hausknecht, Lee-Fay Low, Kate O'Loughlin, Justin McNab, and Lindy Clemson, "Older Adults' Self-Perceptions of Aging and Being Older: A Scoping Review," *Gerontologist* 60, no. 7 (2020): e524–e534. For evidence that positive self-perceptions of aging correspond to living longer, see, for example, Becca R. Levy, Martin D. Slade, Suzanne R. Kunkel, and Stanislav V. Kasl, "Longevity Increased by Positive Self-Perceptions of Aging," *Journal of Personality and Social Psychology* 83, no. 2 (2002): 261–70.

10. For foundational work on bodywork, lifestyle choices, and ways of thinking about conforming to notions of beauty, see Erving Goffman, *Interaction Ritual: Essays in Face-to-Face Behavior* (Aldine Transaction, 1967); Mike Featherstone, *Consumer Culture and Postmodernism* (Sage, 2007).

4. MOTIVATION

1. See the following review of the literature on athletic identity, which indicates that having a strong athletic identity creates resilience and enhances one's abilities to strategize but also increases the risk of depression and other detrimental health conditions, particularly among those who endure serious injury: Bianca R. Edison, Melissa A. Christino, and Katherine H. Rizzone, "Athletic Identity in Youth

Athletes: A Systematic Review of the Literature," *International Journal of Environmental Research and Public Health* 18, no. 14 (2021): 7331–49.

2. Laurel S. Morris, Mora M. Grehl, Sarah B. Rutter, Marishka Mehta, and Margaret L. Westwater, "On What Motivates Us: A Detailed Review of Intrinsic vs. Extrinsic Motivation," *Psychological Medicine* (2022): 1–16. See also Richard M. Ryan and Edward L. Deci, "Intrinsic and Extrinsic Motivations: Classic Definitions and New Directions," *Contemporary Educational Psychology* 25, no. 1 (2000): 54–67; Robert Vallerand, "Intrinsic and Extrinsic Motivation in Sport and Physical Activity: A Review and a Look at the Future," in *Handbook of Sport Psychology*, ed. Gershon Tenenbaum and Robert C. Eklund (Wiley, 2007), 59–83.

3. For more about the negative impact of forced retirement, see Leonardo Martins Barbosa, Bárbara Monteiro, and Sheila Giardini Murta, "Retirement Adjustment Predictors: A Systematic Review," *Work, Aging and Retirement* 2, no. 2 (2016): 262–80. For more about the challenges associated with athletic retirement, see Carrie Esopenko, Josephine R. Coury, Elizabeth M. Pieroth, James M. Noble, David P. Trofa, and Thomas S. Bottiglieri, "The Psychological Burden of Retirement from Sport," *Current Sports Medicine Reports* 19, no. 10 (2020): 430–37; Michelle P. Silver, "Adaptation to Athletic Retirement and Perceptions About Aging: A Qualitative Study of Retired Olympic Athletes," *Journal of Aging and Physical Activity* 29, no. 5 (2021): 828–42; Michelle P. Silver, *Retirement and Its Discontents: Why We Won't Stop Working, Even If We Can* (Columbia University Press, 2018).

4. For more on willpower, see Roy Baumeister and Kathleen Vohs, "Willpower, Choice, and Self-Control," in *Time and Decision: Economic and Psychological Perspectives on Intertemporal Choice*, ed. George Loewenstein, Daniel Read, and Roy Baumeister (Russell Sage Foundation, 2003), 201–16. See also Roy Baumeister, Dianne Tice, and Kathleen Vohs, "The Strength Model of Self-Regulation: Conclusions from the Second Decade of Willpower Research," *Perspectives on Psychological Science* 13, no. 2 (2018): 141–45.

5. Roy Baumeister and John Tierney, *Willpower* (Penguin, 2011).

6. Christiaan G. Abildso, Shay M. Daily, M. Renée Umstattd Meyer, Cynthia K. Perry, and Amy Eyler, "Prevalence of Meeting Aerobic, Muscle-Strengthening, and Combined Physical Activity Guidelines During Leisure Time Among Adults, by Rural-Urban Classification

and Region—United States, 2020," *Morbidity and Mortality Weekly Report* 72 (2023): 85–89. See also Nancy A. Dasso, "How Is Exercise Different from Physical Activity? A Concept Analysis," *Nursing Forum* 54, no. 1 (January 2019): 45–52.

7. For a review of the literature on grit in sports, see Danielle Cormier, Leah J. Ferguson, Nancy C. Gyurcsik, Jennifer Briere, John G. H. Dunn, and Kent C. Kowalski, "Grit in Sport: A Scoping Review," *International Review of Sport and Exercise Psychology* 17, no. 1 (2024): 1–38.

8. Fighting is part of the culture in hockey and sometimes referred to as Rule 46. According to Rule 46 in the National Hockey League (NHL) rulebook, fighting is permitted and it is generally up to referees to determine when a fight occurs and even then, whether and what sort of penalty might be applied if the fight is inappropriate. See, for example, National Hockey League, Official Rules 2024–2025, https://media.nhl.com/site/asset/public/ext/2024-25/2024-25Rules.pdf.

9. Alcoholics Anonymous (AA) started in 1929 as a twelve-step program to help treat alcoholism. By the 1970s, around the time Max connected with it, AA had over one million members. In 1953, Narcotics Anonymous (NA) received permission to use basic principles of AA in its own program.

10. Penelope Lockwood, Jordan M. Jordan, and Ziva Kunda, "Motivation by Positive or Negative Role Models: Regulatory Focus Determines Who Will Best Inspire Us," *Journal of Personality and Social Psychology* 83, no. 4 (2002): 854–64. See also Tory Higgins and Orit Tykocinski, "Self-Discrepancies and Biographical Memory: Personality and Cognition at the Level of Psychological Situation," *Personality and Social Psychology Bulletin* 18, no. 5 (1992): 527–35.

11. For an important book on trauma and healing, see Bessel van der Kolk, *The Body Keeps the Score: Brain, Mind, and Body in the Healing of Trauma* (Penguin, 2014).

12. For reviews of the literature on persistent pain, see Jodie Maccarrone, Ashley Stripling, Julia Iannucci, and Barry Nierenberg, "Exposure to Trauma, PTSD, and Persistent Pain in Older Adults: A Systematic Review," *Aggression and Violent Behavior* 57 (2021): 1359–1789; Fiona J. Clay, Wendy L. Watson, Stuart V. Newstead, and Roderick J. McClure, "A Systematic Review of Early Prognostic Factors for Persistent Pain Following Acute Orthopedic Trauma," *Pain Research and Management* 17, no. 1 (2012): 35–44.

13. For a systematic review of over fifty studies of the concept of resilience in sport, see Christopher Bryan, Deirdre E. O'Shea, and Tadhg Macintyre, "Stressing the Relevance of Resilience: A Systematic Review of Resilience Across the Domains of Sport and Work," *International Review of Sport and Exercise Psychology* 12, no. 1 (2019): 70–111.

14. For insight into the rich literature regarding the U-shaped curve of happiness over time, see Nancy L. Galambos, Harvey J. Krahn, Matthew D. Johnson, and Margie E. Lachman, "The U Shape of Happiness Across the Life Course: Expanding the Discussion," *Perspectives on Psychological Science* 15, no. 4 (2020): 898–912. See also Felix Bittmann, "Beyond the U-Shape: Mapping the Functional Form Between Age and Life Satisfaction for 81 Countries Utilizing a Cluster Procedure," *Journal of Happiness Studies* 22, no. 5 (2021): 2343–59; David G. Blanchflower, "Is Happiness U-Shaped Everywhere? Age and Subjective Well-Being in 145 Countries," *Journal of Population Economics* 34, no. 2 (2021): 575–624; Laura L. Carstensen, Derek M. Isaacowitz, and Susan Turk Charles, "Taking Time Seriously: A Theory of Socioemotional Selectivity," *American Psychologist* 54, no. 3 (1999): 165–81.

15. According to the U.S. Centers for Disease Control and Prevention (CDC), 21 percent of adults have chronic pain and nearly 7 percent experience high-impact pain that substantially reduces their ability to engage in daily activities. See Richard Nahin, Termeh Feinberg, Flavia P. Kapos, and Gregory W. Terman, "Estimated Rates of Incident and Persistent Chronic Pain Among US Adults, 2019–2020," *JAMA Network Open* 6, no. 5 (2023): e2313563. Over 30 percent of adults age sixty-five and over experience persistent chronic pain. For more information, see Carla E. Zelaya, James M. Dahlhamer, Jacqueline W. Lucas, and Eric M. Connor, "Chronic Pain and High-Impact Chronic Pain Among U.S. Adults, 2019," *National Center for Health Statistics Data Brief*, no. 390 (November 2020): 1–8.

5. RESILIENCE

1. For critical discussion and theorizing on the notions of bodywork as well as corporeality and sociology of the body, see Chris Shilling, *The Body and Social Theory* (Sage, 2012).

2. Women have longer life expectancy compared to men. See, for example, Y. Liu, A. Arai, K. Kanda, R. B. Lee, J. Glasser, and H. Tamashiro, "Gender Equality and the Global Gender Gap in Life Expectancy: An Exploratory Analysis of 152 Countries," *International Journal of Health Policy and Management* 11, no. 10 (2022): 2110–18.

3. For more evidence of the relationship between widowhood and health, see Deborah Carr and Susan Bodnar-Deren, "Gender, Aging and Widowhood," in *International Handbook of Population Aging*, ed. Peter Ulhenberg (Springer, 2009), 705–27. For more on the experience of widowhood, see Deborah van den Hoonaard, *The Widowed Self: The Older Woman's Journey Through Widowhood* (Wilfrid Laurier University Press, 2001).

4. Evidence suggests that depression can linger well past five years after the death of a spouse for many women. See, for example, Christina Blanner Kristiansen, Jesper Nørgaard Kjær, Peter Hjorth, Kjeld Andersen, and A. Matthew Prina, "The Association of Time Since Spousal Loss and Depression in Widowhood: A Systematic Review and Meta-Analysis," *Social Psychiatry and Psychiatric Epidemiology* 54 (2019): 781–92. For more on health among widows, see the rich set of articles included in the following review: Anne Lise Holm, Astrid Karin Berland, and Elisabeth Severinsson, "Factors That Influence the Health of Older Widows and Widowers: A Systematic Review of Quantitative Research," *Nursing Open* 6, no. 2 (2019): 591–611.

5. Nuestra Belleza México is a national beauty pageant in Mexico that has more recently been renamed the Mexicana Universal.

6. The typical cost for an emergency room (ER) visit in the United States is around $1,110 per day. The dollar amount varies by location and time, and much of the cost is a result of a combination of direct-care costs and the facility or triage fee. See Marc Roemer, "Costs of Treat-and -Release Emergency Department Visits in the United States, 2021," Healthcare Cost and Utilization Project Statistical Brief #311, Agency for Healthcare Research and Quality, Rockville, MD, 2024, https://hcup-us.ahrq.gov/reports/statbriefs/sb311-ED-visit-costs-2021.pdf.

7. For foundational work on ways the aging body can be seen as threatening to identity, see Peter Oberg, "Images Versus Experience of the Aging Body," in *Aging Bodies: Images and Everyday Experience*, ed. Christopher A. Faircloth (Altamira, 2003), 103–39.

8. See Emmanuelle Tulle, *Ageing, the Body and Social Change: Running in Later Life* (Springer, 2008); Mike Featherstone and Bryan S. Turner, "Body & Society: An Introduction," *Body & Society* 1, no. 1 (1995): 1–12.

6. OPTIMISM

1. For more on the experiences of people living with impairment, see Katie Aubrecht, Christine Kelly, and Carla Rice, *The Aging-Disability Nexus* (University of British Columbia Press, 2020); Tom Shakespeare, *Disability: The Basics* (Routledge, 2017); Alice Wong, *Disability Visibility: First-Person Stories from the Twenty-First Century* (Vintage, 2020); Leah Lakshmi Piepzna-Samarasinha, *The Future Is Disabled: Prophecies, Love Notes and Mourning Songs* (Arsenal Pulp, 2022).

2. For more on optimism and ways of thinking about this concept, see Charles S. Carver, Michael F. Scheier, and Suzanne C. Segerstrom, "Optimism," *Clinical Psychology Review* 30, no. 7 (2010): 879–89. See also Johanna Basten-Gunther, Madelon Peters, and Stefan Lautenbach, "Optimism and the Experience of Pain: A Systematic Review," *Behavioral Medicine* 45, no. 4 (2019): 323–39.

3. For more on stigma among people living with disability, see Sara Green, Christine Davis, Elana Karshmer, Pete Marsh, and Benjamin Straight, "Living Stigma: The Impact of Labeling, Stereotyping, Separation, Status Loss, and Discrimination in the Lives of Individuals with Disabilities and Their Families," *Sociological Inquiry* 75, no. 2 (2005): 197–215.

4. For eloquent writings to help change thinking about stigma, disability, and access, see Cassandra Hartblay, "Disability Expertise: Claiming Disability Anthropology," *Current Anthropology* 61, no. S21 (2020): S26–S36. See also Sanjeev V. Thomas and Aparna Nair, "Confronting the Stigma of Epilepsy," *Annals of Indian Academy of Neurology* 14, no. 3 (2011): 158–63; Tanya Titchkosky, *The Question of Access: Disability, Space, Meaning* (University of Toronto Press, 2011).

5. For a number of recommended works on intimacy later in life and living apart together (LAT) relationships, see Sofie Ghazanfareeon Karlsson and Klas Borell, "Intimacy and Autonomy, Gender and Ageing: Living Apart Together," in *Intimacy in Later Life*, ed. Kate Davidson and Graham Fennell (Routledge, 2017), 1–18; Jenny de Jong Gierveld,

"Intra-Couple Caregiving of Older Adults Living Apart Together: Commitment and Independence," *Canadian Journal on Aging/La Revue canadienne du vieillissement* 34, no. 3 (2015): 356–65.

6. To rethink collective understandings of access, disability, and public space, see Tanya Titchkosky, *The Question of Access: Disability, Space, Meaning* (University of Toronto Press, 2011).

7. Pedro J. Teixeira, Eliana V. Carraça, David Markland, Marlene N. Silva, and Richard M. Ryan, "Exercise, Physical Activity, and Self-Determination Theory: A Systematic Review," *International Journal of Behavioral Nutrition and Physical Activity* 9, no. 1 (2012): 1–30.

8. For more on self-determination theory, see Abraham H. Maslow, "A Theory of Human Motivation," *Psychological Review* 50, no. 4 (1943): 370–96; Abraham H. Maslow, *Toward a Psychology of Being* (Van Nostrand, 1962).

7. COMMITMENT

1. For relevant literature that illustrates the pervasiveness of challenges associated with being a homosexual athlete, see Luca Rollè, Erika Cazzini, Fabrizio Santoniccolo, and Tommaso Trombetta, "Homonegativity and Sport: A Systematic Review of the Literature," *Journal of Gay & Lesbian Social Services* 34, no. 1 (2022): 86–111.

2. For a thorough account of the literature on athletic retirement and the challenges associated with athletic retirement, see Paula Voorheis, Michelle P. Silver, and Josie Consonni, "Adaptation to Life After Sport for Retired Athletes: A Scoping Review of Existing Reviews and Programs," *PLOS One* 18, no. 9 (2022): e0291683.

3. Notable books for the history and context of the HIV/AIDS crisis from a North American perspective include Randy Shilts, *The Band Played On: Politics, People, and the AIDS Epidemic* (Souvenir, 2011); Susan Sontag, *AIDS and Its Metaphors* (Picador, 1989).

4. Felipe enjoys mentioning the celebrities of his era: Rock Hudson was one of the most popular movie stars of his time and among the first celebrities to die of AIDS-related complications. Cazuza and Renato Russo were both acclaimed Brazilian singers and songwriters who died in their thirties due to complications from AIDS.

5. For a thoughtful read on relationships between masculinity and sports, see Michael A. Messner, *Power at Play: Sports and the Problem of Masculinity* (Beacon, 1995).

8. RULES FOR THE ENDGAME

1. In the United States, most adults spend 9.5 hours per day engaged in sedentary behavior and get no exercise on a typical day. For additional information and evidence, see Charles E. Matthews, Susan A. Carlson, Pedro F. Saint-Maurice et al., "Sedentary Behavior in U.S. Adults," *Medicine & Science in Sports & Exercise* 53, no. 12 (2021): 2512–19.

2. Less than 50 percent of U.S. adults meet the Centers for Disease Control and Prevention (CDC) recommendation for 150 minutes of aerobics and two days of strength training weekly. See Christopher G. Abildso, S. Michael Daily, Melissa R. U. Meyer, Christine K. Perry, and Andrea Eyler, "Prevalence of Meeting Aerobic, Muscle-Strengthening, and Combined Physical Activity Guidelines During Leisure Time Among Adults, by Rural-Urban Classification and Region—United States, 2020," *American Journal of Transplantation* 23, no. 3 (2023): 443–46.

3. For foundational ideas behind disengagement theory, see Elaine Cumming and William Earl Henry, *Growing Old* (Basic, 1961). Other ideas, such as modernization theory, follow a similar logic to disengagement theory and suggest more specifically that the emergence of new technology pushes mature adults out of positions of power and prestige, rendering them unable to compete effectively and out of date. For more on modernization theory, see Ernest Watson Burgess, *Aging in Western Societies* (University of Chicago Press, 1960).

4. Activity theory was offered as a counterinterpretation to disengagement theory in 1972 by Bruce W. Lemon, Vern L. Bengtson, and James A. Peterson, "An Exploration of the Activity Theory of Aging: Activity Types and Life Satisfaction Among In-Movers to a Retirement Community," *Journal of Gerontology* 27 (1972): 511–23. They suggested that maintaining higher levels of physical activity later in life is critical to greater life satisfaction. For insights regarding theoretical work that aims to incorporate contextual environmental factors that affect the aging experiences, see Eva Kahana, "A Congruence Model of Person-Environment Interaction" in *Aging and the Environment: Theoretical*

Approaches, ed. Mortimer P. Lawton, Paul G. Windley, and Thomas O. Byerts (Springer, 1982), 97–121.

5. Continuity theory was first proposed by Robert Atchley, who developed his ideas in a series of writings, two of the most prominent include Robert C. Atchley, "A Continuity Theory of Normal Aging," *Gerontologist* 29 (1989): 183–90; Robert C. Atchley, *Continuity and Adaptation in Aging* (Johns Hopkins University Press, 1999).

6. For an in-depth contextualization of the role sports can play in fostering social change, see Douglas Hartmann, *Midnight Basketball: Race, Sports, and Neoliberal Social Policy* (University of Chicago Press, 2016).

7. For the foundational work on age stratification theory, see Matilda White Riley, Marilyn Johnson, and Anne Foner, *Aging and Society: A Sociology of Age Stratification* (Russell Sage Foundation, 1972).

8. Oxidation occurs when an atom, molecule, or ion loses one or more electrons in a chemical reaction. The oxidative stress theory of aging suggests that age-related functional losses are the result of the accumulation of reactive oxygen and nitrogen species. See, for example, Ilaria Liguori, Gennaro Russo, Francesco Curcio et al., "Oxidative Stress, Aging, and Diseases," *Clinical Interventions in Aging* (2018): 757–72.

METHODOLOGICAL APPENDIX

1. See, for example, Sharon R. Kaufman, *The Ageless Self: Sources of Meaning in Late Life* (University of Wisconsin Press, 1986), which examines how people age sixty-five and over interpret aging. Through expressions of a sense of self that is ageless, Kaufman presents continuity in the sense of self. On page 6 of her book, Kaufman suggests that "the voices of individual old people can tell us much about the experience of being old."

2. Since the passage of the Social Security Act in 1935, the age sixty-five has served as a magic number indicating older adulthood and the potential transition to retirement. It is important to note that this age has no particular biological meaning and that what it means to be a certain age, or to be a mature adult, for that matter, has different meanings over time and for different individuals. For more on cross-cultural understandings of age, see Samanta Tannistha, *Cross-Cultural and Cross-Disciplinary Perspectives in Social Gerontology* (Springer, 2016);

Helaine Selin, *Aging Across Cultures: Growing Old in the Non-Western World* (Springer, 2021).

3. For important work on the final stages of life, see Julia Velten, *Extraordinary Forms of Aging: Life Narratives of Centenarians and Children with Progeria* (Columbia University Press, 2022). For a cultural-philosophical critique about the potentials and vulnerabilities of later life, see Hanne Laceulle, *Aging and Self-Realization* (Columbia University Press, 2018).

4. Norman K. Denzin and Yvonna S. Lincoln, *The SAGE Handbook of Qualitative Research* (Sage, 2011).

5. For an indispensable description of narrative gerontology, see Katie de Medeiros, *Narrative Gerontology in Research and Practice* (Springer, 2014). See also Gary Kenyon, Ernst Bohlmeijer, and William L. Randall, *Storying Later Life: Issues, Investigations, and Interventions in Narrative Gerontology* (Oxford University Press, 2010).

6. Janet Z. Giele and Glen H. Elder, *Methods of Life Course Research: Qualitative and Quantitative Approaches* (Sage, 1998); Victor W. Marshall and Margaret M. Mueller, "Theoretical Roots of the Life-Course Perspective," *Social Dynamics of the Life Course* (2003): 3–32.

7. Relevant work was published in Michelle P. Silver, "An Inquiry into Self-Identification with Retirement," *Journal of Women & Aging* 29, no. 4 (2016): 1–12. Another study that introduced ideas relevant for this book is Michelle P. Silver, "Adaptation to Athletic Retirement and Perceptions About Aging," *Journal of Aging and Physical Activity* 29, no. 5 (2021): 1–16.

8. De Medeiros, *Narrative Gerontology*. See also Michael Huberman and Matthew B. Miles, *The Qualitative Researcher's Companion* (Sage, 2002); Johnny Saldaña, *The Coding Manual for Qualitative Researchers* (Sage, 2015); Catherine Kohler Riessman, *Narrative Methods for the Human Sciences* (Sage, 2008).

9. See Robert Atkinson, *The Gift of Stories: Practical and Spiritual Applications of Autobiography, Life Stories, and Personal Mythmaking* (Greenwood, 1995).

INDEX

AA. *See* Alcoholics Anonymous
AAI. *See* Active Aging Index
able-bodied, 59
abusive behaviors, 86
ACSM. *See* American College of
    Sports Medicine
active aging, 28
Active Aging Index (AAI), 13
activities of daily living (ADLs), 23,
    137, 149
activity theory, 188, 226n4
adaptation, embracing, 183
addiction, 86, 96–97, 98; to
    exercise, 99, 101; to painkillers,
    30, 88, 95
ADLs. *See* activities of daily living
adopted children, 133–34
adulthood: agility in, 59; early, 43.
    See also mature adults/adulthood
advanced age, 7
adversity, bouncing back from, 101
aerobics, 62, 80, 93
Aerobics (book), 21
Africa, 19
age: advanced, 7; biological, 79;
    functional, 78–79; happiness

increased with, 104–5; middle,
    sandwich generation and,
    125; peak performance of, 2;
    physiological, 78; psychological,
    78; social, 78; subjective, 79–80.
    See also chronological age
age dysmorphia, 79
ageism, 15
ageless aging, 8–11
agency, 78, 205
age stratification theory, 189
agility, 102, 108; in adulthood,
    59; aging with, 2, 4–7, 54, 180,
    199–200; maintaining, 51
aging: active, 28; ageless, 8–11; with
    agility, 2, 4–7, 54, 180, 199–200;
    antiaging lifestyles, 71; antiaging
    products, 192; embodied, 181;
    health and, 6; judgments on,
    15; luck and, 124; natural signs
    of, 66; "normal," 187; as not for
    wimps, 176–79; perceptions of,
    4, 12–14, 63–68, 105, 171, 180; as
    privilege, 111–14; reflections of,
    191–93; sexuality and, 69; stages
    of, 6; stereotypes about, 13;

aging (*continued*)
strategic, 77–81, 83; subjective, 9;
successful, 57, 78; for women, 63.
See also specific topics
aging body, dissatisfaction with, 71
AHA. *See* American Heart
Association
aids: assistive devices, 127, 140, 151;
mobility, 140
AIDS, 32, 167–68, 170, 177, 225n3,
225n4
alcohol, 95
Alcoholics Anonymous (AA),
96–99, 221n9
AMA. *See* American Medical
Association
American College of Sports
Medicine (ACSM), 21, 186
American Dream, 110, 124
American Heart Association
(AHA), 21, 216n18
American Medical Association
(AMA), 186
Anand. *See* optimism
ancient Greeks, 186
Angelou, Maya, 180, 199
animals, 145–46, 148
anorexia, 39
antiaging: lifestyles, 71; products, 192
anxiety, social, 99
Aristotle, 19
Asha (service dog), 145, 148
Ashe, Arthur, 133, 169
assisted-living facilities, 2
assistive devices, 127, 140, 151
"athlete dies twice," 89–91
athlete's mentality, 189–91
athletic identity, 55, 87–89, 219n1
athleticism, 84

atrophy, 130
attractiveness, physical, 26
Auschwitz concentration camp, 61
Australia, 45

baby boomers, 27, 61
Band Played On, The (Shilts), 225n3
Barbie dolls, 27
Barcelona Games, 217n1
bashert (soulmate), 68
basic intentional movement, 118
Bay Area, 140, 142
beauty: Hollywood ideals of, 73;
identity and, 64; importance
of, 64; mature bodies and, 8–9;
representation of, 80; Western
ideals of, 74; youthful, 8–9, 73, 74
behavior: abusive, 86; habits and,
194–95
beliefs, cultural, 206
belonging, 154
benign paroxysmal positional
vertigo, 120
Biggest Loser, The (TV show), 118
biological age, 79
biomedical manifestations of
corporeality, 131
biomedical models of disease, 5,
77–78
birthdays, milestone, 13
blood pressure, 72, 117, 122, 128
body, 68–69; changes for women,
25–26; changes in, 24–27;
dissatisfaction with, 71; idealized,
24–27; ideal type, 26–27;
"more than a body," 148–50;
out-of-body experience, 161;
"plasticized," 82
body control, 51

body dysmorphic disorder, 41
body shaming, 11
body work, 9, 11, 82
Bollywood, 27
brain: habits and, 194; prefrontal
cortex, 92
Brazil, 32, 157, 159, 164
breast augmentation surgery, 64–66
Buddhism, 19, 37, 44
bulimia, 39
bumps in the road, 94–97
burdens, 138–40
burnout, 40–45

California, 12, 58–60, 73, 75, 83, 140,
142
Canada, 86, 89, 208
cancer, 37
cardiovascular disease, 216n18
Catholicism, 113, 117, 119–20
Cazuza, 168, 225n4
CDC. *See* Centers for Disease
Control and Prevention
cells, declining function of, 7
Centers for Disease Control and
Prevention (CDC), 22–23, 93,
186, 222n15, 226n2
change: in body, 24–27; embracing,
183; habit, 193–96; physical, 25
children, 113–14, 159; adopted, 133–34;
grandchildren, 64; reliance of,
119; toddlers, 6
China, 19
choices, lifestyle, 71, 82, 142
cholesterol, 9
Christianity, 135, 160, 177. *See also*
Catholicism
chronic conditions, 22–23
chronic disease, 3, 7, 10

chronic pain, 3, 105, 156, 173, 202,
222n15
chronological age, 1, 78–80, 124,
219n9; labels and, 6; milestone
birthdays, 13
clavicle fracture, 88
Cold War, 62
Comaneci, Nadia, 217n4
commitment, 32, 156–57, 166–69;
aging as not for wimps, 176–79;
committed athlete and, 160–63;
"everyone is replaceable" and,
163–65; living younger and,
170–73; selfish athlete and,
158–60; timing and, 174–76
committed athlete, 160–63
Common Era, 19
community: disability, 150;
engagement, 36; gay, 166–68, 171;
values, 29
compassion, 155; of animals, 146
competition, 87, 162
competitive drive, 183
concentration, 161
confidence, 29–30, 57–59; body
and, 68–69; doubt and, 81–84;
friendship and, 74–77; invisibility
and, 72–74; "The Luckiest
Generation" and, 60–62;
perceptions of aging and, 63–68;
strategic aging and, 77–81;
unconventionality and, 69–71
congenital conditions, 11
Connie. *See* focus
constructivism, 203–4
consumer marketing, 218n5
continuity theory, 188, 227n5
control: body, 51; cosmetic surgery
and, 82; self-, 92, 94

conversation, 156
cooking, 45–46
corporeality, 3, 131, 206
corrective self-care, 71
cosmetic surgery, 57, 71; breast
    augmentation, 64–66; control
    and, 82; for nose, 64
COVID-19 pandemic, 106, 125, 127,
    145, 150; life expectancy during,
    209; loneliness and, 175; online
    exercise classes during, 67;
    World War II and, 37
critical gerontology, 130, 218n5
cultural beliefs, 206
cultural norms, 83
cultural revolution (1960s), 27
cumulative trauma, 100

dancing, 166
Dark Ages, 19–20
Darwin, Charles, 20
data analysis, 208–9
Davis, Sammy, Jr., 156
death, 83, 203; "athlete dies twice,"
    89–91; chronic conditions and,
    23; euthanasia and, 54; fear of,
    155; grieving and, 113; physical
    inactivity and, 186; premature, 11
dementia, 140
demographic transitions, 216n22
depersonalization, 41
depression, 117, 122, 129, 131, 202;
    athletic identity and, 219n1;
    sedentary lifestyle and, 22;
    widowhood and, 119, 223n4
desexualization, 74
desire, sexual, 69
developmental timing, 205
diabetes, 142, 202

diet, 169, 202
disability, 105; community, 150;
    people with, 146–47
disc compression, 72
discipline, 92
discomfort, habits and, 195
discrimination, ageism as, 15
disease: biomedical models of, 5,
    77–78; cardiovascular, 216n18;
    chronic, 3, 7, 10
disengagement theory, 187, 226n3
disgust, 192
disordered eating, 39
dissatisfaction, with aging body, 71
distraction, 92
distrust, 192
divorced families, 116
dizziness. See vertigo
DNA, 79
dolls, Barbie, 27
double attraction, 60
double back flip, 217n4
doubt, 81–84
drugs, 9, 115, 123; medications, 103,
    122, 129, 131; methamphetamine,
    95; painkillers, 30, 88, 95

early adulthood, 43
early self-monitoring technology,
    140
eating: disordered, 39; of forbidden
    foods, 41. See also food
economics, 136–37, 153
economic status, 10
education, physical, 20
Egypt, 19
elder-care home, 144
elder-care plans, 2
elite athletes. See specific topics

embodied aging, 181

embodiment, 3, 27, 206

emergency room (ER), 128, 223n6

emotional pressure, 38

endgame, rules for, 32, 180–81; athlete's mentality and, 189–91; guidelines from interviewees, 196–98; habit change and, 193–96; living longer and healthier, 182–85; reflections of aging and, 191–93; time is what you make of it, 185–89

engagement: community, 36; disengagement theory, 187, 226n3; of mature adults, 13; with movement, 56

epigenetics, 3–4, 206

ER. *See* emergency room

erectile dysfunction, 91

"ethnic," looking less, 64

European Union, 146

euthanasia, 54

"everyone is replaceable," 163–65

exercise. *See specific topics*

exercise addiction, 99, 101

exercise classes, online, 67, 150–52

expedient lifestyle therapeutics, 71

external (extrinsic) motivation, 92

fairness, 15

falls, 127–28, 130, 141

families: divorced, 116; Jewish, 60–62

fantasizing, 69

fat clubs, 26

fatigue, 43, 195

fear, 177; of death, 155; as motivator, 97

Felipe. *See* commitment

female gymnasts, 217n4

feminism, 25–26

fertility rate: in Brazil, 159; in India, 133; in Japan, 36, 47; in United States, 114

fighting, 221n8

Fiji, 26

film, mature characters in, 6

financial stability, 124

fine motor skills, 104

fitness, 10; collective lack of, 24; movement, 21

flexibility, 53–56

focus, 29, 33; burnout and, 40–45; flexibility and, 53–56; learning to skip, 48–51; listening closely and, 51–52; patience and, 38–40; recalibration for, 45–48; self-, 76; on winning, 34–37

food, 135, 202; cooking and, 45–46; disordered eating and, 39; forbidden, 41; new associations with, 46; plant-based, 169; rationing of, 112

forbidden foods, eating of, 41

fountain of youth, 4

free love movement, 59

friendships, 73, 74–77

functional age, 78–79

functional mobility, 152, 181

gay community, 166–68, 171

gay-related immune deficiency (GRID), 167

Germany, 145, 146–47, 208

gerontology, 6–7, 182, 187–88; critical, 130, 218n5; functional age and, 79; narrative, 204

GI Bill. *See* Servicemen's Readjustment Act of 1944

globalization, 23
global life expectancy, 1
goals: physical, 87; small movement,
    194
grandchildren, 64
gray hair, 8, 25, 70, 72, 80
Great Depression, 60, 205
Greeks, ancient, 186
GRID. *See* gay-related immune
    deficiency
grief/grieving, 113, 144, 177
grit, 94, 109
grooming, 58
gym memberships, 80
gymnastics, 29, 34, 36–37, 40–43,
    48; eating disorders and, 39;
    emotional pressure and, 38;
    female gymnasts, 217n4; routines,
    33; training sessions, 35; World
    Artistic Gymnastics, 35
*Gymnastik für die Jugend (Gymnastics
    for the Youth)*, 216n20

habits: brain and, 194; changing,
    193–96; discomfort and, 195;
    motivation for, 194
hair: gray, 8, 25, 70, 72, 80;
    menopause and, 72
Han, Friedrich, 20
happiness: increased with age, 104–5;
    youthfulness and, 65
health, 213n4; aging and, 6; lived
    experiences and, 5; marriage and,
    119; mental, 5, 136; optimism and,
    144; physical, 5, 136; public, 187
health care, costs of, 2, 23
hearing, 7
heart attacks, 103, 118
high-quality performance, 190

Hillel (Rabbi), 57, 84
hindsight, 142
Hinduism, 19, 136, 141, 145, 151
Hippocrates, 186
Hiroshima, 37
historical time and place, 205
HIV, 167–69, 225n3. *See also* AIDS
hockey, 30, 85–90, 95–98, 104–5,
    221n8
Hollywood ideals of beauty, 73
Holocaust survivors, 61
home photography, 71
homosexuality, 166–67, 178
horses, therapy, 145, 147
Hudson, Rock, 168, 225n4
humility, 174
humor, 151
hygiene movement, 20

ideal body type, 26–27
idealized body, 24–27
identity, 111, 164, 169; athletic, 55,
    87–89, 219n1; beauty and, 64;
    erasing, 64; lifestyle choices and,
    82; multiple, 157; vertigo and,
    120–23
impotence, sexual, 91
independence, 4, 13, 102, 140
India, 26–27, 31, 133
industrial revolution, 20
inertia, 129
infrastructure, sports, 17
injuries, 90, 95–96; clavicle fracture,
    88; traumatic, 100; wrist fracture,
    34, 40, 44
injustice, 44
intentional movement, basic, 118
internal (intrinsic) motivation, 92
interview style and setting, 207–8

intimacy, 77
invisibility, 72–74
ippon, 174

Jamaica, 26
Janice. *See* confidence
Japan, 34, 46, 186, 208; fertility rate
in, 36, 47; temari in, 55; traveling
to, 36–37; women in, 42
Jazzercise, 62, 80
Jewish families, 60–62
Johnson, Earvin "Magic," 169
judgments, on aging, 15
judo, 160–61, 164, 169, 174

Kahn, Robert, 77–78
Kaufman, Sharon R., 227n1
Keep America Beautiful campaign
(1970s), 99
kindness, of animals, 146
Kotelko, Olga, 18
Kübler-Ross, Elisabeth, 110, 131

LAT. *See* living alone together
later-life transitions, 204
legacy, 52
leukemia, 37
Life (magazine), 60
life-course perspective, 204
life-course trajectories, 204
life expectancy: during COVID-19,
209; global, 1
life experience, 201
life satisfaction, 77, 187
life stories, 204
lifestyle choices, 71, 82, 142
listening closely, 51–52
literature, mature characters in, 6
lived experiences, health and, 5

living alone together (LAT),
31, 150
living in pain, 100–102
living younger, 170–73
loneliness, 150, 175
long-term attachments, 85
Los Angeles, 12, 58–60, 75, 83
loss: learning to cope with,
178; muscle, 130; of organ
functioning, 7, 192; resilience
and, 114–17; of tissue, 192; of
weight, 118
love, 73
luck: aging and, 124; optimism and,
136–38
"Luckiest Generation, The,"
60–62

malnutrition, 130
Mandela, Nelson, 85, 108
marginalization, 172
marriage, 63–64, 119
masculinity, 91, 168
Maslow, Abraham H., 154
mature adults/adulthood, 50, 80, 87,
105, 108–9; bodies, 6, 8–9; body
work and, 9; engagement of, 13;
in India, 133; sedentary lifestyle
and, 23; transition into, 3
mature characters, 6
mature models, 27
Max. *See* motivation
maximal oxygen consumption, 18,
216n18
mechanical maintenance, 82
medications, 103, 122, 129, 131
memory, 43
men, 26; attention from, 82; physical
activity and, 22

menopause, 25, 72–73, 75, 76–77
menstrual cycle, 72
mental health, 5, 136. *See also*
    depression
mentality, of athlete, 189–91
methamphetamine, 95
methodology, 203–6
Mexicana Universal, 223n5
Mexico, 30, 110–12, 114, 223n5
middle age, sandwich generation
    and, 125
midlife crisis, 140–45
milestone birthdays, 13
Ministry of Health, Labor, and
    Welfare (Japan), 186
mobility: aids, 140; falls and, 127–28;
    functional, 152, 181; issues, 3;
    physical, 56
modernization theory, 226n3
"more than a body," 148–50
mortality rates, 9
motherhood, 48, 63–64
motivation, 30, 85–86; "athlete dies
    twice," 89–91; athletic identity
    and, 87–89; bumps in the road
    and, 94–97; for exercise, 67;
    external (extrinsic), 92; for
    habits, 194; internal (intrinsic),
    92; living in pain and, 100–102;
    negative role models and,
    97–100; recovery and, 102–7;
    sports and, 107–9; willpower
    and, 91–94
mourning, 41
movement: basic intentional, 118;
    engagement with, 56; physical,
    20, 183, 189, 191–92, 199; small
    movement goals, 194
multiple chronic conditions, 23

multiple identities, 157
muscle loss, 130

NA. *See* Narcotics Anonymous
Nagasaki, 37
Narcotics Anonymous (NA), 96,
    98–99, 221n9
narrative gerontology, 204
National Hockey League (NHL),
    221n8
Nazism, 60
negative role models, 97–100, 109,
    181, 182, 184
neglect, 47, 86
nerve problems, 130
neural pathways, 161
new routines, 195
New Year's resolutions, 93
New York City Marathon, 18
NHL. *See* National Hockey League
nonurban regions, 17
"normal" aging, 187
nose, cosmetic surgery for, 64
nourishment, 154
Nuestra Belleza México, 223n5

Old Testament, 19
Olympic Games, 3, 17, 19, 35, 160,
    217n1; time and, 12; Tokyo, 37
online exercise classes, 67, 150–52
optimism, 31, 133–35; burdens and,
    138–40; exercise as religion and,
    151–55; luck and, 136–38; midlife
    crisis and, 140–43; "more than a
    body" and, 148–50; practice for,
    144–48
organ functioning, loss of, 7, 192
osteoporosis, 72
out-of-body experience, 161

oxidative stress theory, 192, 227n8
oxygen, maximal consumption of,
216n18

pain, 89–90, 95, 104, 195, 210;
chronic, 105, 156, 173, 202, 222n15;
cosmetic surgery and, 66; living
in, 100–102; pushing through, 43,
156; swimming and, 169
painkillers, addiction to, 30, 88, 95
paramedics, for falls, 128
parents, neglect by, 47, 86
passion, 94, 109
patience, 38–40
patient, role of, 118
people with disabilities, 146–47
perception: of aging, 4, 12–14, 63–68,
105, 171, 180; self-perception, 132;
of time, 8, 12–14
perfectionism, 54
performance, 91
perseverance, 94
pessimism, 143–44
pharmaceutical drugs. See drugs
Phelps, Michael, 16
photography, home, 71
physical activity, 10, 22
physical attractiveness, 26
physical change, 25
physical education, 20
physical goals, 87
physical health, 5, 136
physical inactivity, 186
physical intimacy, 77
physical literacy, 183, 186
physical mobility, 56
physical movement, 20, 183, 189,
191–92, 199
physical training, 19–20

physiological age, 78
Pilates, 136
place, historical, 205
plant-based foods, 169
"plasticized body," 82
plus-size models, 27
polio, 135, 202
Ponce de León, Juan, 8
popular culture, 69, 73
post-traumatic stress disorder
(PTSD), 218n5
posture, 178
"powering through," 95
prefrontal cortex, 92
premature deaths, 11
pressure: blood, 72, 117, 122, 128;
emotional, 38; for youthfulness,
70–71
privilege, 185; aging as, 111–14;
exercise and, 123–24
psychological age, 78
PTSD. See post-traumatic stress
disorder
public action, 150
public assistance, 119
public health, 187

qualitative research, 203
quality of life, 13, 188
quick fix, 126–29

railroads, 12
rationing, of food, 112
recalibration, for focus, 45–48
recovery, 102–7
regular exercise, 182
religion, 75–76, 86; Catholicism, 113,
117, 119–20; Christianity, 135, 160,
177; exercise as, 151–55

Renaissance, 20

resentment, 48, 116, 143

resilience, 30–31, 87, 100–101, 110, 131–32; aging as privilege, 111–14; "exercise is not for the poor," 123–24; identity vertigo and, 120–23; loss and, 114–17; quick fix and, 126–29; sandwich generation and, 125–26; somatic thinking and, 117–20; "use it or lose it," 129–30

resistance training, 130

retirement, 89, 162–64, 175–76, 188

risk, avoiding, 74

role models: lack of, 90; negative, 97–100, 109, 181, 182, 184

romance, 80

Roman Empire, 19

romantic desires, 69

Roosevelt, Eleanor, 33, 53

routines: gymnastics, 33; new, 195

Rowe, John, 77–78

Rubens, Peter Paul, 26

Rule 46 (in NHL), 95, 221n8

Russo, Renato, 168, 225n4

safety, 154

Samoa, 26

sandwich generation, 125–26

San Francisco, 140, 142

sarcopenia, 72, 130

satisfaction: dissatisfaction with aging body, 71; life, 77, 187

Scrooge (fictional character), 6

sedatives, 95

sedentary lifestyle, 3, 7, 120, 129, 182, 184; depression and, 22; mature adults and, 23; premature deaths and, 11; in United States, 22, 24

self-actualization, 154

self-care, corrective, 71

self-control, 92, 94

self-determination theory, 151

self-esteem, 91, 154

self-focus, 76

selfish athlete, 158–60

selfishness, 76, 101, 116

self-medicating, 123

self-perception, 132

self-preservation, 184

self-worth, 55

senescence, 7

senses, declining function of, 7

service animals, 145, 148

Servicemen's Readjustment Act of 1944 (GI Bill), 61

sexuality, 159; desexualization, 74; desire and, 69; homosexuality, 166–67, 178; impotence, 91; sexual partners, 170

Shakespeare, William, 26

shaming, body, 11

shelter, 154

Shilts, Randy, 225n3

shingles, 210–11

sight, 7

Silent Generation, 60–61

slimness, 26

small movement goals, 194

sobriety, 96–97

social age, 78

social anxiety, 99

social class, 10

socialization, 150

social media, 71, 80

Social Security Act (1935), 227n2

social standing, 116

somatic thinking, 117–20

soulmate. See *bashert*

specialization, sport, 16
spine flexibility, 19
sports, 10, 14, 87; fairness and, 15; hockey, 30, 85–90, 95–98, 104–5, 221n8; as influential in society, 190; infrastructure, 17; motivation and, 107–9
sport specialization, 16
stereotypes, about aging, 13
stopwatches, 12
stories, life, 204
strategic aging, 77–81, 83
strength training, 130
stress: oxidative stress theory, 192, 227n8; PTSD, 218n5
stretching, 172
subjective age, 79–80
subjective aging, 9
successful aging, 57, 78
surgery, cosmetic, 57, 64–66, 71, 82
"survival of the fittest," 20
Swedish National Institute of Public Health, 186
swimming, 169, 174, 176
systematic reviews, 215n11

teenagers, 6, 27
telomeres, 79
temari (traditional Japanese folk-art), 55
temptation, 92, 177
therapy horses, 145, 147
thinking, somatic, 117–20
thinness, 26, 39
time, 185–89, 192; historical, 205; passing of, 7; perceptions of, 8, 12–14
timing: commitment and, 174–76; developmental, 205

tissue, loss of, 192
toddlers, 6
Tokyo Olympic Games, 37
trauma: cumulative, 100; PTSD and, 218n5
traumatic injury, 100
travel, 36–37, 55
triglycerides, 9
Tulle-Winton, Emmanuelle, 214n9

unconventionality, 69–71
United Nations (UN), 13
United States, 20, 93, 208; economy of, 60; fertility rates in, 114; fitness movement in, 21; kids playing sports in, 16; sedentary lifestyle in, 22, 24; time in, 12
urbanization, 23
urinary tract infection, 128
"use it or lose it," 129–30
U.S. National Senior Games, 18

values, community, 29
vertigo, 117, 120–23
Victorian Era, 92
Vietnam War, 88–89
vigilance, 58

wars: Cold War, 62; Vietnam War, 88–89; World War II, 20–21, 36–37, 60–61
wasa-ari, 174
wealth, 149; as burden, 139
weight, 41, 58; exercise and, 43; loss of, 118; thinness and, 26, 39
weight lifting, 172
well-being: marriage and, 119; optimism and, 144
Western ideals of beauty, 74

Western medicine, 123
WHO. *See* World Health Organization
"wicked old witch" (fictional character), 6
widowhood, 115–16, 118–20, 129, 223n4
Wilde, Oscar, 1, 28
willpower, 30, 91–94, 99
wimps, aging as not for, 176–79
winning, focus on, 34–37
women, 162; aging for, 63; body changes for, 25–26; friendship with, 73–74; GI Bill and, 61; in Japan, 42; physical activity and, 22; widowhood, 115–16, 118–20, 129, 223n4; workforce participation of, 218n3

work ethics, 29
World Artistic Gymnastics, 35
World Health Organization (WHO), 5, 186
World War II, 20–21, 36–37, 60–61
wrist fracture, 34, 40, 44

young adults, 6
youth, 6; fountain of, 4; recapturing, 171
youthful beauty, 8–9, 73, 74
youthfulness, 64, 171; happiness and, 65; pressures for, 70–71
yuko, 174
Yvonne. *See* resilience

Zumba, 80

GPSR Authorized Representative: Easy Access System Europe, Mustamäe tee
50, 10621 Tallinn, Estonia, gpsr.requests@easproject.com

*9 7 8 0 2 3 1 2 1 9 7 4 7 *